The Starting Gate

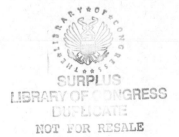

The Starting Gate

Birth Weight and Life Chances

Dalton Conley
Kate W. Strully
Neil G. Bennett

UNIVERSITY OF CALIFORNIA PRESS
Berkeley · Los Angeles · London

University of California Press
Berkeley and Los Angeles, California

University of California Press, Ltd.
London, England

Library of Congress Cataloging-in-Publication Data

Conley, Dalton, 1969–.
　The starting gate : birth weight and life chances /
Dalton Conley, Kate W. Strully, Neil G. Bennett.
　　p.　　cm.
　Includes bibliographical references and index.
　ISBN 0-520-23866-4 (alk. paper).
　ISBN 0-520-23955-5 (pbk. : alk. paper)
　1. Birth weight, Low.　2. Birth weight, Low—
social aspects.　3. Birth weight, Low—Economic
aspects.　4. Social mobility.　I. Strully, Kate W.
(Kate Wetteroth), 1976–　II. Bennett, Neil G.
III. Title.

RJ281.C66　2003
362.1'9892011—dc21　　　　　　　　2002043915

Manufactured in the United States of America
10　09　08　07　06　05　04　03
10　9　8　7　6　5　4　3　2　1

The paper used in this publication meets the minimum
requirements of ANSI/NISO Z39.48-1992(R 1997)
(*Permanence of Paper*). ∞

Contents

Figures

Acknowledgments

We would like to thank all the people, places, and things (not necessarily in that order) that made *The Starting Gate* possible.

Institutional homes for the authors during the tenure of this research project were provided by the Center for Advanced Social Science Research at New York University (Conley and Strully), the New York University Department of Sociology (Conley and Strully), the Sociology Department of the City University of New York Graduate Center (Strully and Bennett), the Baruch School of Public Affairs of the City University of New York (Bennett), the University of California at Berkeley School of Public Health (Conley), and the National Bureau of Economic Research (Bennett). Part of this work was also conducted while two of the authors were at Columbia University's National Center for Children in Poverty (Conley and Bennett). Conley is also indebted to the Institution for Social and Policy Studies at Yale University for support while he was faculty in the Sociology Department there.

Grant support for this project was received from a National Science Foundation CAREER Award; and from the Robert Wood Johnson Foundation, in the form of a Scholar in Health Policy Research Fellowship and an Investigator Award in Health Policy Research.

The authors would like to thank Brian Powell and Jane Mauldon for their helpful reviews at the University of California Press. Other invaluable formal comments were provided by Glenn Firebaugh in his capacity as editor of the *American Sociological Review* (and several anonymous reviewers there); Michael Hughes, editor of the *Journal of Health and Social Behavior* (and associated reviewers); and Ken Land, editor of *Social Biology* (along with anonymous reviewers there, too). More informal but equally valuable suggestions, help, and support were provided by J. Lawrence Aber, Paul Attewell, John Bound, Andrew Clarkwest, and the other participants of Katherine Newman's seminar on social policy at Harvard's Kennedy School of Government; Ismael Fernandez, Jeremy Freese, Bowen Garrett, Arline Geronimus, James House, A. Paula Lantz, Harvey Molotch, Jeff Morenoff, Lincoln Quillian, Barbara Katz Rothman, Karl Schultz, Arland Thorton, Giorgio Topa, Franklin Wilson, Julia Wrigley, and Yu Xie. We are very aware that there are others whom we will remember after this book goes to press, and to them we apologize. We would also like to extend our gratitude to Naomi Scheider at the University of California Press for her editorial assistance and to Sydelle Kramer of the Frances Goldin Literary Agency for her support and legal assistance.

Of course, we each would like to thank our families and friends. Conley and Bennett dedicate this book to their children: Yo and E Jeremijenko-Conley, and Anna and Ari Bennett. Strully dedicates this book to her mother, Diane, who thoughtfully and lovingly raised her own low-birth-weight child.

CHAPTER I

The Baby or the Egg?

Birth Weight and the
Gene-Environment Divide

Where did you come from, baby dear?
Out of the everywhere and into the here.
　George Macdonald, "Baby,"
　Song in *At the Back of the North Wind*

In this book we address two timely and controversial issues. First and most directly, we deal with the causes and consequences of low birth weight, which affects 7 percent of births in the United States.[1] Tiny infants have been surviving in increasing numbers as of late, and our society needs to know the long-term consequences of birth weight for these children.[2] Second, we engage the nature-nurture debate by using the starting point of birth to examine biological and social inheritance. Considering both the biological and the social factors that influence infant health and then looking at the role of infant health on life chances and adult socioeconomic status, we trace, across the following chapters, an intergenerational cycle in which health and socioeconomic status are mutually influential.

The backdrop of this endeavor is the recent resurgence of genetics as an explanation for a wide range of medical and social phenomena. It seems that every week a new medical study emerges announcing that another health risk or behavioral outcome is genetically programmed. Recent findings include genes for breast cancer, left-handedness, anxiety, and homosexuality, to name a few.[3] In a similar vein, a mountain of research has emerged suggesting that our adult health and even our chances for success in life are largely mapped out during infancy. For instance, some researchers have claimed that whether we were breast-fed as infants affects our cognitive ability and school achievement through age 18.[4] Other researchers claim that unborn infants' prenatal environment may account for as much as 50 percent of the variation in intelligence among individuals.[5] However, despite this increasing focus on genetics (nature) and on developmental conditions early in life (nurture), the *interplay between* genetics and environmental factors has been given short shrift in the field of child health and development.

As the determinants of our life course appear to be continually pushed back to the earliest stages of development, we find that nature—genetic factors—appears to win out by default over nurture—environmental explanations. After all, if our future health is largely determined by the time we are born, how could environment play much of a role? The only behavioral/environmental factors that would seem to matter are those of one's forebears, particularly one's mother: did she drink or smoke during pregnancy? Was she over 40 years old at the time of the child's conception? But even these environmental factors have direct chemical or physical links to fetal outcomes. The chemicals in cigarettes damage the fetus.[6] The ova of a woman over 40 have been exposed to more toxins and background radiation than those of a younger woman.[7] More subtle social factors with less obvious physical links, such as racial discrimination or socioeconomic inequality, are neglected in this discourse.

Yet these less obvious environmental factors may play important roles in health and well-being that ought not be ignored. For instance, living in poverty while growing up or during pregnancy is associated with an increased risk of giving birth to a low-birth-weight baby.[8] There are, of course, obvious direct biological links between poverty and health. If poor women have less money with which to buy food, they may have poor diets and thus higher-risk pregnancies.[9] But such direct links do not necessarily tell the whole story. Researchers have also documented that even a mother who is not poor is at an increased risk for giving birth to a low-birth-weight baby if she lives in a neighborhood where most people are poor.[10] Perhaps living in a low-income neighborhood means poor housing conditions, which affect birth weight by increasing exposure to toxins. Or perhaps there are lower levels of social support in poor neighborhoods, which may make it more difficult for a woman to get information about good pregnancy practices or simply may raise her stress level. In either case, there are several indirect paths or mechanisms through which environment may affect biology, and considering only direct chemical or physical environmental effects leaves out a large part of the picture.

Even the social sciences—which would seem positioned to examine the interplay between biology and society—have not been able to fill this gap in our picture of human development. Politics within the social science academy have not been conducive to the study of biology—particularly genetics. Throughout the history of modern social science, *biology* and *genetics* have been dirty words. In fact, the rise to prominence of fields such as social anthropology and sociology at the turn of the twentieth century can largely be seen as an intellectual response to some rather dubious linkages between genetics and social inequality made in the late nineteenth century—for example, connections among blood lines, race, intelligence, and criminality.[11] Such questionable associations continue to plague social science even today. Contemporary researchers Richard Herrnstein and Charles Murray, for example, connect genetics to economic inequality in their book *The Bell Curve,* suggesting that up to 80 percent of intelligence is genetically determined and arguing that—in contemporary society—economic and racial inequality can be almost entirely explained by variations in individuals' inherited ability. Society has become more democratic over the past several hundred years, they argue, implying that genetically determined cognitive ability is now the decisive dividing force in society.[12] Mainstream social scientists, seeking to separate themselves from such arguments, have largely ignored biological and genetic factors in social life for fear of being called biological determinists, leaving the social science discourse over the interactions between biological, genetic, and environmental forces to be dominated by others.

This book seeks to address this overstated separation between nature and nurture by considering how society, biology, and genetics interact with one another across generations. In this endeavor we use low birth weight as a heuristic. In the analysis that follows we consider first the biological, genetic, and social conditions of the previous generation that may lead to a low-birth-weight birth. Then, after establishing the likely causes of low birth weight, we consider the possible long-term social and biological consequences of low birth weight that may determine the next generation's adult success and life conditions. Our results do indeed suggest that biology, genetics, and social conditions are all important for intergenerational patterns of low income and poor health. Using the technique of within-family comparisons, the following analyses show that having a parent who was born low birth weight significantly increases the likelihood that a child will be born low birth weight. Having been born low birth weight him- or herself, a child then faces significantly reduced chances of survival and educational success. But as our within-family comparisons also show, this biological pattern is often dependent on social conditions. The intergenerational transmission of low birth weight and the implications of low birth weight for children's outcomes are partially driven by—and interact with—social factors. By tracing the social and biological conditions of families over long periods, we paint a picture of how social, biological, and genetic factors interact in the case of a particular health outcome—low birth weight.

BIOLOGICAL FACTS OR FICTIONS?

Before moving on to the specific question of birth weight, however, we must further dispel some of the false assumptions frequently made about the relationship among genetics, biology, and environment. Biological researchers often take a reductionist approach to the subject of genetics, failing to recognize the dynamic relationship between genetics and environment. That is, many biologists often assume that genes are a blueprint for an organism, or that an organism—in its essence—can be "reduced" to its genes. Harvard biologist Richard Lewontin summarizes this approach: "The genes in the fertilized egg are said to determine the final state of the organism, while the environment in which development takes place is simply a set of enabling conditions that allow the genes to express themselves, just as an exposed film will produce the image that is imminent in it when it is placed in a chemical developer at the appropriate temperature."[13] A reductionist approach thus assumes that living beings are only the outward manifestation of internal and inherent forces.

Such failure to take into account the classic distinction between genotype (a DNA sequence) and phenotype (the expression of a genetic makeup in a particular environment) leads to several faulty conclusions. Biology and genetics are not one and the same. That someone has a gene for, say, anxiety does not mean that the person will necessarily be nervous. Not every genetic tendency manifests. For such a genetic tendency to express itself, the environment must be conducive. This means that if we took, say, 500 babies with identical genes—all with a tendency toward anxiety—and randomly distributed them in households, some would develop into highly anxious individuals but others would not. Some of these children's environments might be particularly unstable—marked by economic upheaval, crime, or divorce—and in this way, might foster the expression of a genetic tendency toward anxiety.

Other children's homes, however, might not be marked by such disruption, and in these cases the children likely would not end up anxious—their genetic tendencies might be suppressed.

There are also more complex scenarios in which genes may act indirectly and environment may not be so randomly distributed. Indeed it is possible for genes to affect individuals' outcomes by determining their environments. Borrowing an example from Christopher Jencks's discussion of genes and test scores, we can imagine a nation that refuses to send children with red hair to school.[14] In this case the gene that causes red hair can be said to lower test scores, but this does not tell us that children with red hair cannot learn as well as other children. Rather, in this situation, genetics are determining children's environmental opportunities. This is, indeed, an example of a genetic effect, but not the more popular, direct effect discussed above. In this case, it is the indirect mechanism of the social meaning of one's genes that determines their implications. More realistic parallels to this example can be easily found in discriminatory educational and employment practices based on race or sex. If one's skin color or gender means that one cannot attend some schools or hold certain jobs, genetics are determining one's outcomes—but only through the indirect path of the social meaning of genetic characteristics (sex and skin color). Sociologists of science such as Troy Duster have called for a new science of emergent genetics that would address such questions of inequality, genetics, and social opportunity.[15] The classic case given by these sociologists is that a gene for, say, aggression would have very different consequences for a child of privilege than for a child of the ghetto. Because of large differences in their access to resources, aggressiveness might land the first kid in the high-powered boardrooms of corporate America but the kid with few mainstream opportunities for upward mobility in jail.

If we consider further how genes and environment work together, we may quickly note that certain types of genes and certain types of environments go together. That is, people with "advantaged" genes are more likely to end up in an advantaged environment, while those with "disadvantaged" genes are more likely to end up in a disadvantaged environment. According to Christopher Jencks and his colleagues, "Parents with favorable genes tend to have above average cognitive skills. This means that they tend to provide their children with unusually rich home environments. . . . In addition, however, parents with favorable genes usually have genetically advantaged children. These children, thus, end up with a double advantage. They have more than their share of the genes that make for a high IQ score, and they also have more than their share of the environmental advantages that lead to high IQ scores"[16] We can easily imagine how this double advantage could work. There is a great deal of evidence to suggest that positive and warm interactions with children are crucial to intellectual and psychological development.[17] But such warm and positive interactions are not necessarily randomly distributed. There is evidence to suggest, for instance, that parents are more likely to interact with their children in a warm and positive fashion if the child has a pleasant disposition, is responsive, or learns quickly.[18] This means that a child's natural cognitive advantage may lead to more advantageous environmental stimuli. Further, the more interaction this child has with cognitively advantaged parents, the even greater progress this child will make, which may ultimately lead to yet more positive stimuli. Thus, in some cases genes and environment not only commingle but actually build on one another, interacting to create even larger disparities in achievement and well-being. Jencks and his colleagues estimate that, while approximately 45 percent of the variance in IQ scores can be attributed to an individual's genes and their direct consequences, an additional 20 percent of variation must be attributed to this indirect positive association between genes and environment.[19]

WHY EXAMINE BIRTH WEIGHT?

Birth weight provides an excellent example of this confounding of social and biological categories. Birth weight is determined by a whole host of factors, some of which may be genetic but many of which are not. Having a parent who was low birth weight can increase the child's risk of low birth weight, implying a possible genetic inheritance.[20] However, being firstborn or born to a mother who smokes or has a low income can also significantly increase the risk of low birth weight.[21] Regardless of these different factors, once birth weight is determined, it becomes a biological fact, recorded in our medical histories and, in many states, on our birth certificates.

The effects of low birth weight also appear to straddle social and biological divisions. For example, females have a higher chance of being born at low weights than their male counterparts.[22] But, despite this tendency, as well as that of low-birth-weight babies to attain lower levels of education than non-low-birth-weight individuals, females have a higher average educational attainment level than males.[23] Indeed,

56.8 percent of bachelor degrees are now awarded to women, which means that 131 women graduate college for every 100 men.[24] Such a pattern may be the result of multiple factors. Girls may suffer fewer of the biological consequences of their birth weight than boys of similar birth weights. Since the entire birth weight distribution of girls is shifted toward lighter weight, it may be that the cutoff for unhealthy weight is lower for girls than for boys. Alternatively, parents may treat low-birth-weight boys differently than low-birth-weight girls. They may emphasize the vulnerability of a low-birth-weight boy more than the equivalent vulnerability of a low-birth-weight girl—or vice versa. Birth weight is a biological condition, yet it may be caused by and may lead to a series of factors that are genetic, biological (but nongenetic), or social.

There are several additional reasons to examine low birth weight. To begin with, birth weight is a good indicator of infant viability and is easy to measure. Low birth weight is not a disease per se but a reflection of one or more underlying perinatal health issues. A baby may be born low birth weight for several reasons ranging from elevated maternal blood pressure, to poor maternal nutrition, to the prenatal onset of leukemia.[25] Birth weight is also simple to assess because almost everyone knows his or her birth weight, and those who do not usually can check their birth certificates (in many states) or call a parent to find out.

Further, birth weight is an appealing heuristic for examining inheritance, because it measures health right at the "starting gate" of life. That is, since birth weight has many lasting effects on health and well-being throughout childhood and adulthood,[26] it allows us to consider how one's health position at the "starting gate" affects one's later chances for success. Thus, with birth weight as our case study, we can take into account not just the transmission of a biological condition from mother to child but also the transmission of general health status across multiple generations. If a female baby born low birth weight, afflicted during her childhood with the consequences of low birth weight, grows up and has a child of her own, we can consider the transmission of health status from the grandmother to the mother and then from the mother to the grandchild. That is, we can consider how cycles of health are maintained across generations.

Finally, since birth weight displays such intergenerational patterns while straddling the biosocial divide, studying it helps sort out the possible roles of biology, genetics, and society in creating and maintaining inequality. Average birth weights among groups are very sensitive to social inequality, such that African Americans and the poor are at a disproportionate risk of being born low birth weight.[27] Poverty and racism may also heighten the long-term deleterious implications of low birth weight.[28] However, echoing such patterns across social divisions is the clustering of low birth weight within families. Having parents or siblings who were born low birth weight is associated with an increased risk of being born low birth weight,[29] and such within-family clustering may suggest a genetic or biological component to the risk and consequences of birth weight. In short, birth weight is a very rich index with several unique characteristics that may be exploited for intergenerational sociobiological analysis.

Concepts and Measurements of Low Birth Weight

Although interest in prematurity and low birth weight dates back to the end of the nineteenth century, there remain controversial issues regarding their conception and measurement. The earliest concepts of prematurity and inadequate fetal development were based entirely on gestational age. A birth was classified premature if the pregnancy terminated before the completion of its tenth lunar month but after the seventh, which was used as a standard of fetal viability. However, being born early does not necessarily equate to being born underdeveloped physiologically. Also measurement error may arise from irregularity of the menstrual cycle, uncertainty as to the date of last menses, or misinterpretation of uterine bleeding during the first months of pregnancy as menstruation. Because of the imprecision of calculating gestational age (or the expense and complication of calculating it with greater accuracy) and the imperfect correlation between pregnancy duration and fetal development, birth weight became a popular and officially sanctioned measure of immaturity shortly after World War I. It was agreed that some standard of evaluation and comparability was needed. What easier measure than merely weighing the infant at birth? So in 1935 the American Academy of Pediatrics resolved that, for statistical purposes and comparison of results of care, a uniform standard of diagnosis of prematurity is important. A premature infant is one who weighs 2,500 grams (five pounds, eight ounces) or less at birth (not on admission), regardless of the period of gestation. All live-born infants were to be weighed, with evidence of life being heartbeat or breathing.[30]

The substitution of birth weight for maturity measurement, however, does not come without its own sources of error. While it may seem very simple to distinguish between a live birth and a stillbirth, it can actually be quite complicated. Internationally, the definitions of live births vary considerably, leading to sizable differences in the number of births eligible to be diagnosed as premature or low birth weight. In some industrialized countries a birth is considered live if one of two criteria is satisfied—either the infant shows signs of life (i.e., breathing or beating heart), or the fetus is over a certain length of gestation.[31] So, even if an infant is born with no sign of life, it will still be considered a live birth if the gestational cutoff was reached.

International ambiguity in the definition of live births arises from variation in the second criterion for live birth—the gestational cutoff. In most U.S. states, all fetuses over 20 weeks of gestation are potentially live births and thus are included in the assessment of prematurity and low birth weight. However, in several other industrialized countries— including France and England—the gestational cutoff is much higher (28 weeks), significantly reducing the number of births considered live and eligible to be counted as premature or low birth weight.[32] This difference in the definition of live births can have striking implications on rates of low birth weight. The United States' infant mortality rate has traditionally been quite high as compared to other industrialized countries. However, when adjusting for differences in the measurement of birth weight, researchers have found that the U.S. rate is actually lower than those of England, Wales, and France.[33] This means that international differences in the definition of live birth lead to such variation in the reporting of birth weight that the ordering of infant mortality rates can actually fluctuate.

Beyond these questions of what should count as a live birth, there are also problems of measurement surrounding the etiology of low birth weight. A baby may be born abnormally small because she was born too early or because she did not develop adequately in the womb— despite reaching full gestation. In the first case, the baby's small size results from prematurity. In the second case, the baby's small size is a result not of prematurity but of abnormal growth patterns (often called intrauterine growth retardation, or IUGR). As recent technologies such as ossification timing have become available for assessing gestational length more accurately, it has become apparent that prematurity and IUGR can be thought of as distinct phenomena that play different roles in infant health.[34] To the extent that physicians and researchers are sensitive to this distinction and prematurity is registered separately from low birth weight resulting from IUGR, we may see significant changes in rates of low birth weight. Specifically, rates of low birth weight would appear to drop as all those infants born prematurely (with normal fetal growth rates) would no longer be classified as low birth weight. Research also suggests that such a narrowing of the definition of low birth weight would shift race gaps in birth outcomes since black-white differences in rates of premature births are significantly larger than black-white differences in rates of IUGR births.[35] We will examine these questions of race, etiology, and infant health in greater detail in chapters 2 and 4.

Nonetheless, low birth weight is an important predictor of a number of health and developmental outcomes regardless of whether it reflects prematurity or inadequate uterine growth. Each year in the United States, about 250,000 low-birth-weight infants are born. Among this group about a fifth are born of very low birth weight (that is, born weighing less than 1,500 grams).[36] These rates of low birth weight play an important role in determining the infant mortality rate, since death rates of the neonatal period (first month of life) are quite sensitive to birth weight.[37] Among babies born in 1991, the infant mortality rate for those who weighed over 2,500 grams at birth was 3.5 per 1,000; it was 21.8 per 1,000 for babies born weighing between 1,500 and 2,500 grams; while a staggering 296.4 per 1,000 very-low-birth-weight infants died within the first year of life.[38] In fact, in 1991 medical complications associated with low birth weight and preterm delivery were the primary cause of death among black infants and the third leading cause among white infants.[39]

Infant Mortality, Low Birth Weight, and Inequality

During much of the twentieth century, infant mortality steadily declined, largely as a result of reductions in the postneonatal (ages two to twelve months) death rate. This improvement can mostly be attributed to reductions in infectious diseases. As sanitation improved and vaccines were developed, young children were less likely to fall prey to diseases like pneumonia, measles, or tuberculosis. However, between 1960 and 1980 there was an epidemiological shift, and the greatest declines in infant mortality took place in the neonatal stage of life (first month). These declines in mortality were largely a result of new technologies that came on line in neonatal intensive care units, most notably improvements in respirators. Babies who were vulnerable at birth could now be sustained through crucial periods thanks to medical interventions. Indeed, during that 20-year period of rapid technological advances in neonatology, 90 percent of the decline in the neonatal death rate was due to improved birth weight–specific survival rates.[40] That is, the steep drop occurred in the death rate for both low-birth-weight and non-low-birth-weight babies, not in the rate of low birth weight.

Since the 1980s the decline in infant mortality has stagnated because rates of low birth weight have not improved. In fact, the incidence of low birth weight has increased, and there has been little offsetting reduction in birth weight–specific mortality rates.[41] Birth weight is, thus, central to any further decrease in the infant mortality rate. It is precisely the death rates for the neonatal period, which are largely dependent on birth weight, that have not budged.[42] Yet cutting this mortality rate by lowering rates of low birth weight will not be simple. Despite the large improvements in infant health outlined above, the fact of birth weight's sensitivity to social inequality complicates efforts to reduce rates of low birth weight further. Blacks suffer from rates of low birth weight approximately double those for whites. This fact partially explains the vast difference in infant mortality between the two groups as well as the difference in scores on tests of cognitive ability.[43] Low-income parents can also face between two and three times the risk of a low-birth-weight birth compared to high-income parents.[44] Therefore, when seeking to reduce overall rates of low birth weight—and the associated rates of infant mortality—it is necessary to recognize specific social groups and address inequalities in risk.

At the same time, the relationship between birth weight and inequality is not altogether straightforward. Since race differences in low birth weight have been far easier to ascertain than socioeconomic differentials, researchers have had a great deal of trouble sorting out racial and economic factors in low-birth-weight gaps, and results on this topic remain quite mixed. For example, Barbara Starfield and her colleagues find that, for children born to white mothers in the National Longitudinal Survey of Youth (a 1979 survey of 12,686 individuals aged 14 to 21 followed over time) poverty increases the incidence of low birth weight but that for blacks in the sample it makes no difference (though blacks have a higher risk at all socioeconomic levels).[45] In a similar vein, Chiquita Collins and her colleagues find that for Hispanics urban poverty is negatively associated with birth weight only when the mother is Puerto Rican or a U.S.-born member of another subgroup.[46] However, yet another study finds that, among African Americans, family poverty has a powerful effect on the risk of delivering a low-birth-weight baby even after accounting for family and neighborhood demographic characteristics.[47]

In addition, a host of factors associated with income and race may further confound efforts to isolate racial and economic factors in low birth weight. Some are socioeconomic, others behavioral. Among the socioeconomic and demographic factors affecting birth weight are maternal age (women under 20 and over 35 are at a higher risk of delivering an LBW infant), labor force status (working mothers tend to experience greater risk, particularly in occupations that expose women to second-hand smoke), education level (higher education leads to lower rates of low birth weight), parity (firstborns are more often of low birth weight), birth spacing (pregnancies spaced close together are more likely to result in low birth weight), maternal stature (the smaller the mother, the smaller the baby), weight before pregnancy, and weight gain during pregnancy (the lower the mother's initial weight and subsequent weight gain, the lighter the infant at birth). Behavioral factors such as maternal alcohol, cigarette, or drug use have long been known to increase the risk of low birth weight, as has maternal smoking.[48] Many of these factors (such as smoking) are now common knowledge, while others (such as birth order) are not yet well understood.

Nonfatal and Later Life Consequences of LBW

For those children who do survive the first year of life, birth weight (and the compounding effect of certain subsequent social conditions) is a very important predictor of several measures of development. Weight at birth may determine both physical health and psychological conditions within the family. Among animals for which multiple births are the norm, birth weight is a clear determinant of suckling order. The runt of the litter may often wither and die from lack of nourishment for failure to adequately compete with its siblings for access to the mother's teat. If the runt lives, its personality may be quite different from those of its siblings.[49] Even among humans, for whom singleton births are the norm, birth weight may have important psychological dimensions for the development of a child if she or he is labeled fragile, delicate, or sickly.[50] (In fact, the physician in charge of the first premature baby ward in 1898 described low-birth-weight premature babies as *les enfants debiles* ["weak children"] and associated their condition with congenital weakness.[51])

While these labels may end up having psychological or physical causality themselves, more notable are the well-documented physical deficits from which low-birth-weight babies often suffer. By age six and a half, over 40 percent of low-birth-weight infants experience one or more physical or mental handicaps, ranging from cerebral palsy to mental retardation to epilepsy.[52] Preterm and low-birth-weight infants also suffer in their psychological and intellectual development. Holding other factors constant, there is a direct relationship between gestational age at birth and developmental scores in a variety of tests at multiple ages.[53] Some research has shown that at age four and a half years, low-birth-weight children tend to perform poorly on the British ability scales (an IQ-like test).[54] Additionally, more subtle abnormalities, such as visual-motor disability and subnormal development of language comprehension skills, have been detected in as many as 30 percent of low-birth-weight (LBW) babies.[55] Visual recognition memory has been shown to be deficient among LBW infants, implying that they may have greater trouble processing information visually than their non-LBW counterparts.[56] Behavioral disorders have also been found to be more prevalent in LBW children. Studies suggest that at infancy LBW babies fuss and cry more, are less soothable, and tend to change behavioral states more often than non-LBW babies.[57] At older ages, LBW children—particularly boys—exhibit further behavioral problems, ranging from depressive and anxious disorders to hyperactivity and aggressiveness.[58]

Low-birth-weight infants also suffer from much higher rates of illness than normal birth weight infants. On average, low-birth-weight babies experience one to three readmissions during the first year of life for such reasons as lower respiratory infections, gastrointestinal problems, hypertension (high blood pressure), and inner ear infections (otitis media).[59] These early conditions can lead to several longer-lasting conditions. For example, lower respiratory illnesses often lead to shortness of breath when the toddler or young child attempts to participate in play and sports.[60] In fact, one study of children ages one to four documented that 35 percent of surviving low-birth-weight babies were limited in one or more activities of daily living.[61] While the birth weight–specific survival rate has increased dramatically since the 1980s, the rate of dysfunctionalities for the survivors has budged very little.[62] Since contemporary neonatal technologies allow babies to live who 20 years ago would have died, these infants are more likely to demonstrate health and developmental problems for the very fact that they were such marginal survivors.

This troubling situation raises important questions about the long-term prospects of marginal survivors. Each type of dysfunction—neurological, cognitive, behavioral, and physical—can significantly hinder a low-birth-weight child's progress through school and ultimately make it difficult for the child to attain socioeconomic success as an adult. Such lasting effects of low birth weight have only recently begun to receive attention, but evidence collected so far suggests that differences between low-birth-weight and normal-birth-weight children can last well into adulthood. For instance, a group of researchers in Denmark found that the average cognitive functioning (IQ) of 18-year-old male draftees was significantly lower among individuals born low birth weight.[63] Additionally, Maureen Hack and her colleagues, following poor babies born in Cleveland, found that, at age 20, very-low-birth-weight individuals are less likely to have graduated high school and more likely to be chronically ill than normal-birth-weight individuals.[64]

However, since inequality is so strongly tied to the risk of low birth weight, it can be quite difficult to isolate the biological effects of low birth weight. Poverty may interact with the biological condition of low birth weight to create a very poor prognosis for the many low-birth-weight babies who live in poverty. A study by Robert Bradley and his colleagues found that, at age three, only 12 percent of premature babies living in high-risk situations (poverty) functioned at the normal cognitive level—significantly worse than premature babies born to low-risk families.[65] Additionally, poverty may have many of the same deleterious effects as low birth weight on child development (i.e., chronic health problems and intellectual deficits), making it very difficult to sort out whether low birth weight or poverty is to blame for children's conditions.[66]

INHERITANCE OF LOW BIRTH WEIGHT:
SOCIETY OR BIOLOGY?

That a certain trait—biological, social, or other—appears in consecutive generations does not mean that its reproduction is due to genetics or biology. In some instances, inheritance does reduce to genetics, as in the case of eye color. In others, genetic, biological, and cultural factors may come together to create complex patterns. Such appears to be the case in the matter of low birth weight. If a mother was low birth weight (and has had no previous LBW children), her child has a 250 percent greater risk of being low birth weight him- or herself than does a child with a non-low-birth-weight mother (with no previous LBW children); if she was low birth weight and already a had an LBW child, the odds for another child being low birth weight are greater than fifteen times that of a child with a non-LBW mother and normal-birth-weight siblings.[67] For some, this pattern implies genetics. For example, one medical doctor casually noted that she believed there exists a genetic link in the size of babies at birth across generations, since women who were big themselves at birth tend to give birth to big babies. There even appears to be an ethnic component to this genetic inheritance since, the doctor observed, those of Germanic stock tend to display this pattern.[68] However, alternative, nongenetic explanations also abound. For instance, the association may be a result of similar behavior patterns across generations. If a woman's mother smoked during pregnancy, resulting in her being born low birth weight, and the woman herself smoked while carrying her own child, resulting in that child being of low birth weight, as well, this may create the appearance of an intergenerational, *genetic* association between mother's and child's birth weight, when the true association is between grandmother's and mother's pregnancy behavior (in this case, smoking).

Birth weight is indeed a case in which genetics, biology, and society become intimately linked, and existing research presents very little consensus on how to explain the intergenerational transmission of birth weight. Some research has suggested that mothers may indeed transmit low birth weight to their children through their genes. One study has documented that infants with a certain genotype (ALPp*1/*1) for placental alkaline phosphatase (PLAP) were less likely to be born low birth weight than babies who had other genotypes.[69] A study by Jere Behrman and Mark Rosenzweig uses identical twins to factor out genetic variation across mothers and finds that the intergenerational inheritance of low birth weight has a very strong genetic component.[70] When comparing a random sample of births, these authors find a strong relationship between maternal and filial birth weight. But when factoring out genetic differences by comparing births to mothers who are identical twins, they find no association between maternal and filial birth weight. It thus appears that a large part of the maternal-filial association found in the random sample is the result of genetic variation associated with birth weight.

However, other studies have suggested that inheritance may be a result of the environment in which fetuses develop rather than the genes they begin with. Researchers who gathered data from 62 births that resulted from ovum donations found that the donor's (genetic mother's) birth weight had no significant influence on the birth weight of the child from the donated ovum, while the recipient's weight did.[71] Such a finding clearly demonstrates the importance of uterine environment. Interestingly, findings from this study were replicated with horse fetuses. Malnourished horse fetuses were placed in the wombs of either thoroughbred horses (with larger wombs) or regular horses (with smaller wombs). Those fetuses transplanted into thoroughbred horses' wombs were born closer to normal birth weight than the fetuses transplanted into regular horses' wombs, implying that the uterine environment played a crucial role in the fetuses' development.[72] It must be noted, though, that the reliability and generalizability of the results from both these studies is questionable. The study of ovum donors has a small sample that is likely not representative of the larger population, and comparisons between horses and humans are, at best, problematic. Nonetheless, these results do suggest the potential of biological—yet nongenetic—factors in the inheritance of low birth weight.

Behavioral and environmental factors may also be quite important in the inheritance of low birth weight. Since one learns many behaviors from one's parents, poor pregnancy practices—such as smoking, not seeking prenatal care, and having poor nutrition—are likely to be clustered within families and may be learned across generations. This means that behavioral causes of low birth weight may be inherited across generations. Social conditions, particularly poverty, may also create the illusion of a genetic component to low birth weight. Parents' poverty appears to increase the risk of filial low birth weight (although it is unclear whether this association varies across racial and ethnic groups). But poverty at early ages also has negative effects on later educational attainment, job status, and earnings.[73] Therefore, when a low-birth-weight individual who grew up in poverty has a child, there is a higher than average chance that this child will be born into poverty. The social condition of poverty inherited across generations may also be an independent factor behind family patterns of low birth weight.

The Role of the Father

Most of the discussion thus far has explicitly—or implicitly—focused on the behavior, environment, and genes of the mother who bears the infant. But what about the father's contribution to the baby's weight?

Dads would seem to provide the ideal heuristic to identify genetic effects on birth weight: they contribute genes but do not carry the fetus. However, while a paternal effect likely implies a genetic component to birth weight, this is not necessarily so. As with the discussion of mothers above, there still are several alternative explanations that must be noted. Possible confounding effects range from the dynamics of the marriage market to secondhand smoke to environmental toxins. The first possible dynamic that could produce a nongenetic effect on birth weight has to do with assortative mating dynamics. If, for instance, low-birth-weight males tend to marry low-birth-weight females or tend to marry women who have poor nutritional habits, then a paternal association may merely reflect the maternal effects combined with at-risk fathers' tendency to marry mothers of the same ilk.

A second potentially confounding effect could be paternal behavior. Clearly, the father's nutritional status during pregnancy does not matter to the child (except as an indirect, statistical reflection of the mother's). However, some paternal pregnancy behavior may affect the fetus quite directly. Perhaps the most obvious is smoking. A father who smokes while living with his pregnant partner exposes her to secondhand smoke. Secondhand smoke exposure during pregnancy has been suggested as a potential contributing factor to the incidence of low birth weight, though the empirical evidence so far is limited. There is some documentation of an association between paternal smoking and infant birth weight. For instance, Fernando Martinez and his colleagues found birth-weight deficiencies when mothers did not smoke but fathers smoked more than 20 cigarettes a day. It remains unclear, however, whether this effect acts through the secondhand smoke mechanism or rather through teratogenic effects on sperm.[74]

Teratogenesis is indeed another mechanism by which the father could affect the child's birth weight. If a father was exposed to hazardous material, used narcotics (or cigarettes), or was irradiated during the period prior to conception, his spermatoza might have been altered for the worse, affecting the birth weight of the child through some sort of congenital malformation. The literature on paternal effects is sparse as compared to that on maternal forces; nonetheless, there is some evidence to suggest that exposure to certain deleterious substances may affect the genetic makeup of a man's sperm. Until very recently, the guiding paradigm of sperm theory was an "all or nothing" model according to which, if some toxin damaged a sperm, it was out of the game. In other words, given the intense difficulty in and competition for penetration and insemination of the ovum, sperm that were damaged in some way would not be capable of performing and thus would be rendered infertile. However, this paradigm has recently been criticized,[75] and some research has shown that male mice that were exposed to morphine or alcohol sired progeny that had a high rate of birth defects, even when factoring out maternal exposure. Even the grandchildren of these mice demonstrated birth defects, suggesting that mutogenesis can occur from the father's side.[76]

Other evidence indicating the salience of paternal health to birth outcomes includes research that documents a link between paternal occupational exposure to paints, solvents, dyes, and other such materials with an increased incidence of childhood cancer and tumors, spontaneous abortion, and Down syndrome.[77] One study showed that the offspring of men who demonstrated symptoms of exposure to the defoliant Agent Orange during the Vietnam War had twice the incidence of congenital anomalies of veterans without such symptoms.[78] All these studies demonstrate a growing recognition that men's behaviors and environments can affect birth outcomes independently of maternal factors.

However, for such paternal behavior or environment to cause the appearance of genetic inheritance where there is none, the father's action or environment would have to contain an intergenerational flavor. That is, if a father smoked during his spouse's pregnancy and his father smoked, as well, during his own gestational period, then there could be an intergenerational association resulting from social rather than genetic forces. Or teratogenesis must have occurred so that a mutation persists through the generations. The likelihood that such dynamics of consistent exposure or mutation would explain relationships that persist through succeeding generations within the overall population is slight. Since the father's nongenetic effect on the fetus is necessarily less direct than the mother's, it is more difficult to find confounding mechanisms contributed by the father that are so systematic and consistent as to *seem* genetic. Despite nongenetic possibilities, paternal effects on offspring's birth weight remains a useful tool in our efforts to sort out inheritance mechanisms.

MEASUREMENT ERROR: THE CASE OF OBESITY AND EARNINGS

The entanglement of social, biological, and genetic influences is not surprising—processes of inheritance are indeed complicated. However, the confounding of these influences can have dire effects on research results. Failing to explicitly take into account peoples' individual endowments (genetics) or their environments can lead researchers to detect false relationships. Most people, regardless of their political or theoretical inclinations, will admit that individuals vary at least to some degree in their natural abilities and talents. To the extent that such variations are associated with environmental factors (such as income, family structure, or neighborhood), it is easy to confound genetics and environment. For instance, to the extent that one's health endowments vary with income, it can be hard to tell which leads to which. Healthier people can work more hours and thus earn more money. Or people with more money can buy more health-related resources, thus increasing their health. Or people with good health and high earnings may also be greatly motivated, which in turn leads to better health behavior *and* better employment. In many existing studies, associations between these various factors make it very difficult to tell which of the above scenarios is actually taking place. In technical terms, variation in people's ability and genetics is called "endowment heterogeneity," and failing to take into account such heterogeneity can lead to seriously biased results.

Research on obesity and human capital provides some effective examples of this type of bias. Studies have shown that being overweight or obese leads to reduced schooling and wages—at least for white women in the United States.[79] Speculating on mechanisms that may drive this relationship, authors have cited discrimination and work loss due to higher rates of illness and early retirement among overweight individuals.[80] While such a relationship seems plausible, given the emphasis on beauty in our culture and evidence of health problems related to obesity, contrary arguments challenge this sort of explanation strongly. There are numerous claims that low income or poverty causes obesity, particularly for women in highly stratified and industrialized countries like the United States, implying that low wages may be causing obesity rather than vice versa.[81] Equally plausible mechanisms can be imagined for this reverse association. For instance, behavioral factors affecting weight, such as diet and exercise, which vary across class, may be driving a class effect on obesity. Stress related to low socioeconomic status may similarly play a role in obesity via behavioral mechanisms. Most studies of obesity and socioeconomic status have been unable to adequately sort out health and socioeconomic influences; consequently, the direction of causation is often unclear.

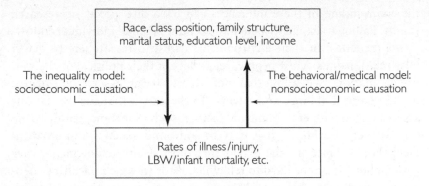

Figure 1.1. The possibility of reverse causation (LBW, low birth weight)

Since many health measures are associated with socioeconomic conditions, this problem of causation is indeed rather widespread in health research. In technical terms, many studies of health and inequality are plagued by the possibility of reverse causation. As indicated with the left-hand arrow in Figure 1.1, it may be the case that socioeconomic status (determined by a host of factors) is leading to poor health (similarly indicated by a number of different factors). However, it may likewise be the case, as indicated with the right-hand arrow in the figure, that poor health is leading to low socioeconomic status.

In addition, there is even another scenario that may explain these associations between weight and socioeconomic status. A third factor, individual endowments, may be responsible for the association between socioeconomic status and obesity. It is possible that individuals with tendencies toward obesity also have tendencies toward low socioeconomic status and that the joining of these two tendencies at the individual level generates the association between obesity and low earnings. In this scenario, we find a spurious effect rather than reverse causation. That is, as outlined in Figure 1.2, we have a third, unobserved factor (individual endowments) causing both biological conditions and socioeconomic status. But, when we cannot measure this third factor, it may appear that socioeconomic status and health are directly linked to one another. In this case, we say the association between socioeconomic status and health is spurious (false). Again, this problem of indeterminate causation is rather widespread in health research since individual endowments are potentially determinants of most health outcomes as well as most measures of economic well-being, and we will encounter this problem again at several points in this book.

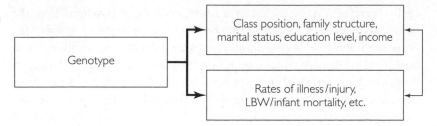

Figure 1.2. The possibility of spurious effects: the genetic model (LBW, low birth weight)

Recent research suggests that this scenario of individual endowments may be very important to the association between obesity and earnings. Susan Avarette and Sanders Korenman find that, when factoring out a portion of individual endowments through sibling comparisons, the negative relationship between body mass and wages is significantly reduced.[82] Jere Behrman and Mark Rosenzweig, factoring out even more variation in individual endowments using identical twin comparisons, find that the negative relationship between body mass and earnings disappears entirely when individual propensities are taken into account.[83] These problems in determining causation are extremely important in our discussion of low birth weight. For example, recent research suggests that individual endowments are indeed a concern with regard to low birth weight and education. Behrman and Rosenzweig, using identical twins to factor out variation in endowments, found that the positive effect of increasing birth weight on schooling was *underestimated* by 50 percent when endowments were not adequately factored out.[84]

This result, however, should not be interpreted as the last word and in fact may overestimate birth weight effects. Although identical twins often seem to be revered as the holy grail of genetics research, there are reasons to believe that they may not be the most reliable subjects—particularly for birth weight research. Identical twins are a unique subset in society and can be exposed to particular dynamics—prenatally and throughout their life courses—that may render their experiences ungeneralizable to the rest of the population. In the case of birth weight, whichever twin occupies a more advantageous uterine position—that is, closer to the placenta and thus closer to maternal nourishment—usually has a much heavier birth weight. Often the smaller of the two twins is born undernourished and in the danger zone of birth weight.[85] Because twins share the same uterus, they are in direct competition with each other for nutrients. Given a finite amount of nutrients that the twins may access, every ounce that one twin gains implies a loss for the other twin. Because of this unique prenatal competition, a difference in birth weight between twins may represent a more serious health disparity than a birth weight difference between two babies that did not share the same womb. This may reduce the generalizability of the results from twins to the larger population. We will return to this issue in chapter 4 when we examine a database of twins.

RESEARCH APPROACH

This book offers a next step in sorting out the complexities of nature and nurture with respect to birth weight and its sequelae. Most epidemiological studies lack adequate information on the medical and socioeconomic history of both parents and thus do not allow us to isolate social and biological influences in the inheritance of life chances. Further, most social science data sets do not have the detailed medical information that would allow us to isolate etiological factors and separate the implications of specific health conditions from general ones. We get around these common limitations by using two data sets: long-term longitudinal data from the Panel Study of Income Dynamics (PSID), and shorter-term longitudinal data from the Matched Multiple Birth Data Set. While not originally designed to address issues of infant morbidity, the PSID is a nationally representative sample of American families starting in 1968. Its advantage lies in being the only data set to our knowledge that has socioeconomic histories of family members along with their birth weight status.

    With this information, we can isolate the effects of each parent's socioeconomic status from his or her biological condition (i.e., birth weight). While the PSID does not have genetic information per se, by combining family medical history information with socioeconomic data, we can indirectly determine if certain intergenerational patterns are a result of genetic, biological, and/or social factors. That is, using within-family comparisons to factor out the genetic contributions of parents, we can examine the pure effects of social factors. While it is true that, except for identical twins, no two children have exactly the same genetic makeup, when we observe socially *systematic* differences in birth outcomes among children from the same family, we may conclude that this is a true social effect. The use of such within-family comparisons allows for greater certainty than has been attained before in the analysis of social factors' impact on birth weight. Likewise, in comparing the educational performances of siblings from the same family, we can isolate the effects of birth weight from other socioeconomic or biological factors.

However, since the PSID does not provide information on specific causes of low birth weight, we cannot be entirely sure that what we observe as birth weight effects are indeed effects purely of birth weight and not either partially or fully reflecting more general health conditions that are associated with birth weight. As mentioned before, there are a number of specific conditions that may lead to low birth weight, ranging from maternal blood conditions to the prenatal onset of leukemia.[86] Or more generally, low birth weight may reflect an overall disposition toward poor health (in the mother, the child, or both). Thus we may be detecting the implications of these conditions in our analysis rather than the implications of birth weight itself. To get around this problem of ambiguous etiologies, we supplement the PSID data with the 1995–1997 Matched Multiple Birth Data Set, which provides information on the pregnancies, fetal deaths, births, and infant deaths in multiple deliveries. Using the twin pairs in this data set, we can factor out almost all the differences in prenatal conditions and varying differences in genetic compositions (depending on whether twins are identical or fraternal)—that is, we can factor out most of the underlying conditions that may be reflected in birth weight effects. Therefore, by exploiting the differences between the twins in this data set, we can be relatively certain that we have isolated the precise impact of size at birth on—in this case—infant mortality.

Using twin pairs, siblings, and cousins, we repeatedly employ family comparison techniques. Within-family comparison provides many advantages over standard statistical techniques. In the latter, randomly selected individuals are compared on the issue of interest, and the researcher attempts to factor out additional systematic variation by including variables in the model that are in some way related to the outcome of interest. Such analyses are sometimes problematic, however, because the researcher can rarely be sure that he or she included all necessary related factors in the analysis.

However, comparing two individuals within the same family (be they twins, siblings, or cousins), rather than randomly selected individuals, greatly reduces the amount of unobserved, systematic variation between individuals and thus reduces the potential for spurious results. Because full siblings, for example, share the same parents, this type of comparison factors out much of the genetic and biological variation that may lead to low birth weight. Parents' genetic makeup will not change between one birth and another, and biological factors that may affect birth weight, such as the size of the womb or the mother's stature, will similarly not change (though the womb may, of course, be different the second or third time around—we take this into consideration). Of course, nontwin siblings share only 50 percent of their genes on average, but for genetic differences between them to generate a spurious association between, say, poverty during the mother's pregnancy and which of the two was born low birth weight, poverty would have to somehow be associated with which genes each child got—a far-fetched possibility. In other words, the 50 percent of genes that siblings do not share is like random background noise and should not bias any causal inference. This ability to factor out genetic and biological variation allows us to be more confident that the social effects that we may find in the following analyses are true social effects, unbiased by unobserved genetic or biological variation.

In addition to factoring out genetic variation, within-family comparisons also allow us to factor out some unobserved variation in environmental factors. If we compare two individuals' risk of low birth weight, one individual living in poverty and the other not, the effect of poverty that we find may be overstated, because these two individuals' households may differ in several subtle ways related to income. However, because individuals in the same family usually grow up in the same household, we reduce this potential for unobserved variation related to environment. Sibling and cousin comparisons, however, are not as effective at reducing environmental variation as they are at reducing genetic and biological variation, because environmental factors are more likely to systematically change between two pregnancies than are potential biological or genetic factors. For instance, it is possible that a mother might relocate between pregnancies due to a loss of income and be exposed to different environmental factors between pregnancies. It is highly improbable that a grown woman will be significantly taller for one pregnancy than the other.

Although the PSID, which we use in the majority of our analyses, provides very rich data for these comparisons, it does not record specific behaviors that may influence birth weight, like smoking, prenatal care, or drinking. Fortunately, however, within-family comparisons help here too. In analyses of a standard sample, there would be no way to factor out behavioral variation, because we would have to include these factors in the model and we do not have data on them. In sibling and cousin comparisons, in contrast, behavioral variation is reduced to a change in behavior that must take place *between* pregnancies. (Behavioral variation is not a concern for our twin comparisons, since these pairs experienced common pregnancies.) So for smoking to bias our results in a sibling or cousin comparison, a mother would have to pick up or quit smoking between two pregnancies. Additionally, for behavioral variation to significantly bias our results, it must vary *systematically* with our factors of interest (e.g., low birth weight and poverty). This means that changes in behaviors like smoking or drinking would have to coincide with changes in income in order for behavior to bias the effect of income. If a woman suffered a loss of income between pregnancies and began to smoke or drink in response to such stress, the positive effect of income on birth weight may be overstated. Alternatively, if a woman increased her income between two pregnancies and began to smoke or drink for this reason (however unlikely), the positive effect of income on birth weight would be understated.

While such scenarios are of course possible, their ability to significantly alter our results is not great. For instance, if a woman smokes in response to stress from loss of income and this raises her risk of a low birth weight birth, smoking is really only a mediating factor in the more important relationship between income and low birth weight. As long as our factors of interest (parental birth weight, poverty, and race) are primary causes and not mediating factors in such scenarios—which is more likely—these types of behavioral factors are of little concern. Thus, while we cannot completely factor out behavioral variation that may influence birth outcomes, we can significantly reduce the possibility of it biasing our results.

There are two other potential sources of unobserved variation that may be issues in our analysis: vulnerable child syndrome and maternal recall bias. Vulnerable child syndrome posits that parents view low-birth-weight children as weaker and more delicate than non-low-birth-weight children and may modify their parenting accordingly. If parents consider their child to be more vulnerable than other children, they may place restrictions on the child's behavior or lower their expectations for the child. In our analyses of the connections between low birth weight and educational attainment and between low birth weight and infant mortality, such a syndrome may be a problem. For instance, if a child's birth weight leads a parent to lower his or her expectations for the child and such lowered expectations cause the child to perform poorly in school, we may find a seemingly direct biological connection between birth weight and educational attainment that is, in truth, indirect and nonbiological. In this scenario, lowered expectations related to birth weight are causing low educational attainment, while birth weight itself is having no direct, biological effect. Sibling and twin comparisons, unfortunately, will not address this potential source of bias, since we will have no way to measure with the PSID or the Matched Multiple Birth Data Set whether parents within the same family treat specific siblings differently based on birth weight. However, while vulnerable child syndrome certainly warrants some attention, it may not be too great a concern, since there is generally little empirical evidence to support this syndrome and any systematic differences in parents' treatment of children based on birth weight seem to be limited only to very early ages (which implies that this may be more of a problem in our analysis of infant mortality than in our analysis of longer-term educational outcomes).[87]

Maternal recall bias, another potential source of unobserved variation, is more applicable to our education analysis and occurs when parents are more likely to remember the low-birth-weight status of a child with educational problems than that of a child without such problems. If two children are born low birth weight but only one has developmental or educational problems in later life, the mother, trying to cognitively reconcile her children's current lives with their births, may be more likely to remember that the child with later problems was low birth weight. That is, problems at birth will form a better cognitive fit with the more "problematic" child than with the other. These hypotheses of maternal recall bias fit within a long theoretical tradition in social psychology that portrays people as cognitive conservatives and posits that people bias their memories to maintain consistency.[88]

In our analysis, this tendency to reduce dissonance may exaggerate a positive relationship between low birth weight and low educational attainment. If mothers are more likely to recall complications at birth when a child's education is also complicated, we may overstate the effect of low birth weight on low educational attainment. However, there are several reasons to doubt the importance of this potential bias. To begin with, there is little empirical evidence suggesting that mothers tend toward such bias. When researchers have compared hospital records to maternal reports of birth weight, they have generally found that mothers can accurately recall their children's birth weights.[89] Also, since the general public is largely unaware of connections between birth weight and educational attainment, it would seem rather unlikely that mothers would feel a strong need to cognitively reconcile their child's birth weight with his or her educational attainment. Further, since the PSID asks people many varied questions at one time, it again seems unlikely that mothers would feel any strong tensions specifically between the information they give about their child's birth weight and that about his or her education.

ORGANIZATION OF THE BOOK

Chapter 2 presents our first statistical analysis. We address the question, Does a historical legacy of low birth weight or a legacy of social disadvantage account for the propensities of African Americans to be born low birth weight? While many scholars share a social approach to the issue, arguing that social and economic factors are of primary importance in the relationship between race and infant health, there is still much debate within this social arena over which of these nonbiological factors matter most. On the other side of the fence, several scholars have proposed genetic explanations for racial differences in birth weight, arguing that infants of different races may "naturally" come in different sizes because of genetic differences between African American and white populations. In this chapter, we try to assess whether the intergenerational transmission of low birth weight is indeed biological or genetic by using grandparent fixed-effects models (or maternal cousin comparisons) to factor out, to a great extent, family socioeconomic circumstances. Our results suggest that accounting for the inheritance of parental low birth weight explains much of the black-white gap in low birth weight. Intergenerational legacies of poor health are indeed important in explaining racial disparities in health.

Chapters 3 and 4 consider intergenerational cycles of low birth weight and low income. In chapter 3, we treat income and parental birth weight as determinants of filial birth weight and use sibling comparisons to sort out the relative contributions of and interactions between social and biological factors. In Chapter 4, we consider how filial birth weight affects life chances—both literally and figuratively. We first use sibling comparisons to examine the roles of filial birth weight and early childhood poverty in educational attainment. We then address whether birth weight effects are a true result of infant size or rather a proxy for other health conditions. Here we use twins to consider the specific role of birth weight in infant mortality. In considering the intergenerational inheritance of low birth weight, poverty, and life chances in these two chapters, we address two related questions: how does the previous generation determine a baby's well-being at birth, and how do these birth conditions determine the baby's life chances? Our results suggest that biological and social factors work and interact with each other in determining birth outcomes, infant mortality, and educational attainment. Analyses from chapter 3 find that maternal income has a significant impact on birth weight for those infants who already face a hereditary risk (i.e., have a low-birth-weight parent). The chapter 4 analyses find that low birth weight dramatically increases the chances that a child will not graduate from high school in a timely fashion, but that incomes at high enough levels may attenuate this biological effect. Using twin comparisons, this chapter also finds that actual weight—not acting as a proxy for other perinatal conditions—affects the risk of infant mortality.

In our final chapter we consider the implications of our results. Here we argue for a redefinition of categories and concepts of risk. Our findings that biological risk is important but that economic resources can also counteract biological effects imply that economic and social resources need to be more effectively targeted at those facing *both* biological and social disadvantage. We consider how practitioners, policy makers, and parents alike may use biological risk categories to focus prevention and intervention efforts. We pay particular attention to the programs and questions surrounding access to medical care, income, and special education.

John Henry, Black Mayors, and Silver Spoons

Race and the Inheritance of Birth Weight

John Henry was a little boy,
No bigger than the palm of your hand,
'Time that boy, he was nine years old
Driving spikes like a man.
Driving spikes like a man.

    Folk song

An important indicator of a society's development is the mortality rate among its infants. Differences between black and white trends in infant mortality in the United States clearly reflect the existence of two societies that are only growing further apart. In 1950, the African American rate of infant mortality (43.9 per 1,000) was more than 1.5 times the white rate (26.8 per 1,000).[1] Almost fifty years later, the likelihood of infant death had decreased for both groups, but black-white differences increased, so that the mortality rate among black infants in 1999 (14.6 per 1,000) was more than twice the rate for white infants (5.8 per 1,000).[2] In other words, despite large improvements in infant mortality over the past half-century, African American rates remain much higher than white rates. Black-white differences in low birth weight are equally wide. The rate of low birth weight among black infants in 1999 (11.3 per 1,000) was more than twice that for white infants (5.0 per 1,000).[3]

Far beyond the first year of life, blacks are faced with higher rates of sickness and death than their white counterparts. As of 1998, risk of death for the black population was at least 1.5 times that for the white population for seven of the ten leading causes of death. The largest difference in risk was found in the category of homicide, in which a black individual was 5.7 times as likely to be murdered as a white individual. The next largest difference was in rates of death from hypertension, with a black individual having 3.8 times the risk of death from this cause. Septicemia, kidney disease, and diabetes similarly presented differential risks for blacks and whites, with blacks facing between 2.4 and 2.7 times the risk of death from these causes.[4]

The result is that blacks on average live significantly fewer years than whites. A black man born in 1999 could expect to live 67.8 years, while a white man born the same year could expect to live 74.6 years—almost a seven-year difference in life expectancy. A black woman born in 1999 could expect to live 74.7 years, while a white woman born that same year could expect to live 79.9 years—a slightly smaller, though still sizable, difference of just over five years.[5] In addition to these differentials in survival, African Americans are also more likely to have their health status become a burden. Among adults, blacks are almost twice as likely as whites to assess their health as fair to poor (15.1 percent versus 8.6 percent), and are more likely than whites to report that a chronic condition limits their activity (15.8 percent versus 13.4 percent).[6]

While race is clearly important to both infant and adult health, there is little consensus over why this is so. Many scholars argue that social factors are of primary importance in the relationship between race and health, while others alternatively suggest that biology and genetics are largely responsible for racial discrepancies in low birth weight. In this chapter we will examine patterns of social and biological inheritance over generations in an effort to reveal the factors underlying race differences in birth outcomes. Our results, based on within-family comparisons, suggest that biological inputs are quite important in explaining race differences in rates of low birth weight. That is, black-white differences in biological legacies of low birth weight appear to explain a substantial part of the gap between black and white rates of low birth weight. But, as we will discuss below, this evidence cannot necessarily be interpreted in a biologically determinist fashion. Rather, we find that the manifestation of biological risk can depend on environmental factors.

A BRIEF CASE STUDY OF HYPERTENSION: INTERGENERATIONAL CYCLES

One of this book's main assumptions is that race, class, society, and biology can be most effectively sorted out by expanding the time horizons of most studies and considering the impact of prior generations. That is, if we take into account the influence of parents and grand-parents, we can more effectively factor out the indirect influences that may be entangled in a particular outcome before a study or an individual life begins. Of course, in studying infant health, the maternal impact cannot be ignored and has been addressed in most studies. At the starting gate of life, biological and social impacts on the infant are largely mediated through the mother. We propose, however, that the mother's adult health is similarly affected by the biology and social conditions of her mother and that, to understand the relative impacts of biology and society, it is necessary to consider inheritance across more than two generations.

Findings surrounding hypertension are a very good example of how consideration of multiple generations may reveal complex processes. As noted above, blacks face almost four times the risk of death from hypertension as whites.[7] Explanations for this differential stir a debate over biological and social influences that is very similar to that which we encounter in discussions of low birth weight. For instance, on the social side of the fence, socioeconomic status may explain blacks' elevated risk of hypertension. Stress related to financial, family, and neighborhood (e.g., crime) problems disproportionately affect blacks and may increase the likelihood of hypertension. Similarly, low socioeconomic status places constraints on health-promoting behavior (e.g., diet and exercise) and thus may increase the likelihood of hypertension via behavioral mechanisms.[8] Other authors who propose social explanations for hypertension rates have suggested that racism is of key concern.[9] Experiences of racial discrimination (particularly for blacks with dark skin) have been shown to be associated with elevated rates of hypertension.[10]

In contrast to these models focusing on quality of life and stress, some researchers have found that African American infants have higher heart rates at birth than white infants, regardless of socioeconomic status. Such authors have used these results to suggest that an inherent biological condition may explain part of African Americans' tendencies toward hypertension.[11] If racial differences are apparent at birth, it is usually assumed to be logically problematic to explain such disparities with social conditions. Infants are at the beginning of life and thus have not had time to accumulate the biological marks of social position that most social explanations of disease rely on. Because no infant has experienced, for instance, socioeconomic status or racial discrimination, it is often assumed that biology rather than society is to blame for conditions at birth. That is, without the infant having experienced social factors, it is assumed that society cannot be causing disease.

Presented with these contrasting biological and social explanations of hypertension, we can consider how intergenerational models may bridge the dichotomy in perspectives. A mother has lived out her life in society, and thus her social position, stress, and other environmental conditions may leave biological marks on her (such as hypertension) that may then affect her baby while in utero. A baby, affected by her mother's hypertension, may then exhibit a higher than normal heart rate at birth. At this point, the biological trait of heart rate may be attributed to the mother's social position. However, if this baby grows up under the same social conditions as her mother and develops the same condition of hypertension in adulthood, is this case of hypertension the result of a health condition at birth or of social conditions in later life? It is quite hard to tell. In addition, if this individual with hypertension has a baby with a higher than normal heart rate, interpretation of the factors underlying this third generation's health becomes even more complicated. In this situation, there appears to be a biological inheritance of heart rate linked to hypertension, but the role of social conditions in the mother's (and grandmother's) hypertension still remains a very important factor.

The disadvantaged position of African Americans across generations can quickly confound social and biological elements. In this example the first case of a high heart rate at birth was a result of the mother's social conditions, but from that point on, the relative social and biological contributions to adult hypertension were quite obscure. Our topic of low birth weight presents many similar intergenerational dilemmas that may be addressed by expanding the time limits of our analysis.

COMPETING SOCIAL EXPLANATIONS OF LOW BIRTH WEIGHT

Most of the current debates over race and health address the question of whether and how race may be explained in terms of class—that is, whether the relatively disadvantaged position of blacks is a result of a disproportionate risk of being in poverty or a result of noneconomic aspects of race.

Race and Class

Black-white differences in socioeconomic status can be found at almost all ages. Tracing the lives of two imaginary children, one black and one white, we find a notable disparity in life chances. To begin with, child one, born to an African American mother, has three times the chance of living in poverty before the age of six as child two, born to a white mother.[12] Children one and two are also likely living in different family situations. Child one faces a 69.3 percent chance of being born to a single mother, while child two faces a 21.9 percent chance.[13] Child one and her fellow black students have about an 85 percent chance of obtaining at least a high school diploma; child two and her fellow white students, about an 88 percent chance. There are, however, large differences related to race in the quality of elementary and high school education, such that many schools with majorities of black students lack crucial resources like textbooks and qualified teachers. These disparities in quality mean that, despite similar amounts of education, blacks often bring fewer basic skills to the labor market than whites.[14] Indeed, child one is more than twice as likely as child two to become unemployed. And when employed, child one is also approximately twice as likely as child two to end up in a service industry that offers lower pay, fewer benefits, and less stability than the professional or managerial positions that child two could more easily secure.[15]

The race-class debate attempts to explain why these gaps persist. In his book *The Declining Significance of Race* William Julius Wilson argues that, thanks largely to the civil rights movements of the 1960s, overt racial oppression has largely been eliminated in the economic sphere. However, instead of blatant discrimination, Wilson argues, socioeconomic (i.e., class) differences between blacks and whites maintain blacks' disadvantaged position. As Wilson writes in his book's opening sentence, "Race relations in America have undergone fundamental changes in recent years, so much so that now the life chances of individual blacks have more to do with their economic class position rather than their day-to-day interactions with whites."[16] This argument enjoys some statistical support. For instance, there has been increased occupational mobility for African Americans across and within generations. And when class is taken into account, African Americans demonstrate significant advantages over their white counterparts on certain educational measures (namely high school completion).[17] Yet there is

also evidence to suggest that race still matters in, for example, predicting earnings and wealth for given educational levels.[18]

Beyond such divergent statistics, authors have also argued that race
maintains important symbolic power in society, even if overt discrimination is now illegal. Cornell West, in his book *Race Matters*, offers several examples of his personal experiences with discrimination in order
to demonstrate the continued significance of race. For instance, West
recounts multiple empty taxis passing him by, only to stop for white
people further up the street, and his being the victim of unfounded
police harassment. West contextualizes these experiences by reminding
us that blacks are seen as not conforming to mainstream (read: white)
society and, thus, to be black in the United States is to be associated
with social problems.[19] According to this argument, even if race can be
statistically factored out of many models, its importance in individual
and social well-being can still remain salient.

Race, Class, and Health

Empirical results with respect to race and health are mixed.[20] In one
study, 77 percent of race differences in premature births were explained
by socioeconomic status.[21] Other studies have found more modest
effects. Nancy Moss and Karen Carver, for instance, found that income
and socioeconomic variables explained only about 20 percent of black-
white differences in low birth weight.[22] However, despite different sizes
of class effects, neither study is able to wholly explain race differences.
Lending some support to the critiques of purely economic models, it
seems that race continues to matter to at least some degree, regardless
of the power of class effects. Indeed, almost all studies that factor out
socioeconomic status are plagued with some level of unexplained racial
variance. Race does not seem to be entirely reducible to class with
regard to health.

Variations in *how* race affects health across income levels also point
to the continued significance of race. Most studies suggest that racial
disparities in health are wider among higher socioeconomic groups.
For instance, there is evidence to suggest that racial variation in birth
weight is greater in higher-income areas than in lower-income areas.[23]
Similar evidence regarding education and pregnancy has revealed that,
within a certain range of attainment, education protects black women
from pregnancy and birth complications less than it does white
women.[24] These tendencies imply, rather ironically, that African Amer-

icans who are "making it" financially are lagging even further behind their white counterparts than African Americans who are less well-off. It is unclear why this is so. Socioeconomic status is often more complicated than many assume, and certain resources may have multiple meanings depending on context. As an example, a college education may be helpful in getting a job in a predominantly white suburb that offers mostly administrative and managerial positions, while the same college degree may be of only limited use in a predominantly African American inner city offering mostly low-grade service jobs. Such outcomes may, however, depend not so much on context as on the inadequacy of existing methods of measurement. Subtle socioeconomic differences between blacks and whites may slip past crude statistical tools, leaving the appearance of independent race effects.

Measuring Socioeconomic Status

Our ability to statistically sort out race and class can be no more effective than our ability to accurately measure these two categories. If certain aspects of one's class background are not captured with existing measures, the effect of such class factors will appear to be unexplained variance when in fact they should be attributed to socioeconomic status. The three measures that usually constitute socioeconomic status in existing studies are education, occupation, and income. These are not necessarily bad measures. They are powerful, explaining a significant amount of variation in well-being and life chances, and are relatively easy to measure. Education is usually measured in terms of years of formal schooling; occupation is often categorized by prestige. Income is usually measured in real dollars. However, there are likely more than three factors that constitute class status, so the frequent use of these measures may mean that we are missing a large part of the picture.

One component of class that receives little attention but likely has a significant influence on health is wealth. Assets in the forms of savings, stocks and bonds, businesses, and real estate can play a crucial role in one's economic well-being. Wealth can provide a nest egg that protects a family during periods of income instability (brought about by sudden events like illness or unemployment). Wealth can also allow one to make investments that will bring later monetary returns. For instance, assets can be used to invest in higher education that leads to higher income in the future.

Evidence suggests that wealth plays a sizable role in race differences in life chances. In 1998 white families with the median net worth of $81,700 had a median nest egg of financial wealth totaling $37,600. In the same year, African American families with the median net worth of $10,000 had a median nest egg totaling only $1,200. Breaking these numbers down, we see that for every dollar of white financial wealth there are three cents of black financial wealth.[25] Further analysis has suggested that these differences have important implications in the long run. For instance, factoring out multiple forms of socioeconomic resources—including parental wealth—reveals a significant black net advantage in educational attainment and income. When net worth is taken into account, blacks are 2.67 times more likely to complete high school and tend to earn $1.42 more per hour than their white counterparts.[26] More complete measures of class that take into account the wealth of the prior generation not only reduce racial disparities but also may actually reverse them on some measures.

The relationship between wealth and health has received relatively little attention; however, evidence suggests that wealth does matter with respect to health. One study found that family assets were strongly related to mortality even when factoring out the effects of education and first occupation.[27] Studies in Britain have similarly shown that home and car ownership is associated with lower mortality.[28] While these studies break crucial ground in further understanding the relationship between health and wealth, they do not necessarily imply a causal relationship and may be plagued specifically by reverse causation. While these studies suggest that wealth makes one healthier, it may also be that better health makes it easier for one to accumulate wealth. A healthier person can work more hours, generating more money for investing, or may have a more future-oriented perspective that fosters investing and wealth accumulation.

There are several reasons why wealth may be important to a baby's risk of low birth weight. For instance, wealth's role in providing financial stability and security may be particularly relevant to birth outcomes. Evidence suggests that income instability and stress related to financial well-being during pregnancy increase the risk of unhealthy birth outcomes.[29] Since wealth can be drawn upon in cases of income loss such as unemployment, assets may provide an additional resource to white women that allows them to avoid financial fluctuations that can have harmful effects on babies. Additionally, wealth may be particularly important in analyses of low birth weight because wealth is often inherited rather than earned. Direct transfers, such as bequests of assets, have been estimated to account for approximately 46 percent of household wealth in the United States.[30] Since wealth is much more stable within families and across generations than is income, occupation, or education, it may be crucial in maintaining the conditions that contribute to family patterns of low birth weight. Even if there is a significant difference between mothers' and daughters' incomes, the inheritance of assets will likely remain stable across generations, implying that even in the face of income fluctuations, black and white socioeconomic differences may remain relatively stable. Despite all of this, however, our preliminary analyses revealed no association between wealth and low birth weight.

Other class factors that are rarely measured, though they may be important in health disparities, are residential segregation and housing conditions. In the United States these two issues are intimately linked to race. In 1999, 33 percent of whites in the Census Bureau's metropolitan statistical areas, as compared with 64 percent of blacks in these same areas, lived in central cities. Meanwhile, 36 percent of blacks and 67 percent of whites in metropolitan statistical areas lived in suburbs.[31] This spatial concentration of minorities in inner cities has repeatedly been shown to be associated with higher rates of low birth weight and mortality.[32] However, the mechanisms behind such connections are poorly understood. For example, it is plausible that simply the predominance of certain individual-level characteristics explains connections between segregation and poor infant health. Women living in highly segregated areas are more likely to have low incomes, be unmarried, and be less educated than those living in less segregated areas,[33] and these characteristics have all been shown to increase the risk of unhealthy birth outcomes. A recent study by Ingrid Ellen offers some empirical support for this individual-level explanation. According to Ellen, factoring out the marital status and education of the mother reduces the risk of a low-birth-weight birth for black women living in segregated areas by between 22 and 62 percent.[34]

However, an alternative and slightly more complicated mechanism that may also drive the connection between segregation and health is differential access to resources across neighborhoods. Studies have found that low-income minority neighborhoods have fewer pharmacies, restaurants, banks, and specialty stores as compared to high-income neighborhoods, which ultimately means that minority women have to travel farther, sometimes paying more, to get what they need.[35]

The quality of housing may also be an issue with segregation since minority families are more likely to live in areas with abandoned buildings or in apartments with multiple inadequacies.[36] Such evidence suggests that because health-promoting resources are relatively scarce in minority neighborhoods, it may be more difficult for minorities to stay healthy. Such access-based explanations remind us of how economic resources can take on various meanings depending on the situation. A black dollar and a white dollar do not necessarily grant access to resources with equal power if neighborhood characteristics are unequal. While black and white individuals may receive similar scores on commonly used socioeconomic scales, those scores may have different implications if the context of those resources varies significantly.

The connection between segregation and health may also be a question of behavior. If minorities in highly segregated areas engage in less healthy activities than those in nonsegregated areas, different behavioral profiles may be to blame for health disparities. Ingrid Ellen offers some empirical support for this explanation as well. When tobacco and alcohol use during pregnancy and the use of prenatal care are factored out, the risk of low birth weight for black women in segregated areas falls by up to 55 percent.[37] It should be noted, though, that such behavioral factors are not necessarily playing a primary causal role. Behavioral differences across neighborhoods may be mediating rather than actually replacing the effects of segregation. Most of one's behaviors are not arbitrary but are influenced by those around one. Thus, a segregated neighborhood context may increase the chances that a pregnant woman will engage in an unhealthy behavior, like smoking, by blocking the flow of information about its risks. In this case, behavioral differences are connecting segregation to health, rather than entirely accounting for the effects of segregation on health—as would be the case if smokers selectively migrated into racially segregated neighborhoods of other smokers.

A final issue with the way we measure class that may be particularly salient for low birth weight is the timing of class measurement. As mentioned in chapter 1, most evidence suggests that early childhood—and even prenatal socioeconomic conditions—have a lasting effect on life chances and health.[38] Most studies of low birth weight examine or socioeconomic status around the time of pregnancy, thus failing to consider whether the mother was in poverty during her early childhood. Research of low birth weight may therefore not fully account for the socioeconomic conditions that might have the most deleterious effect on health.

It may be early poverty, which is rarely measured, that really matters in health outcomes. This could be important for explaining race differences in health, since middle-class minorities are more likely to have been poor during their childhoods than their white counterparts. A recent study by Mary Patillo-McCoy and her colleagues found that in 1994 middle-class blacks were four times as likely as middle-class whites to have been poor as adolescents.[39] Such different rates of upward mobility mean that, by the time African American mothers enter a study, cumulative health damages that are not captured by current class status may be affecting birth outcomes. The timing of poverty may also speak to the larger racial differences we find in higher as compared to lower socioeconomic groups. If a larger number of middle-class black mothers than white mothers spent their childhoods in poverty, we may note a larger racial disparity in higher-income groups that is due to past economic situations that are *not* being studied.

Beyond Class: The Symbolic Meaning of Race and Discrimination

There is a great deal of debate not over the existence of blacks' socioeconomic disadvantage but over whether such disadvantage means that race can be reduced to class, as Wilson suggests. As West outlines in his book *Race Matters*, race can have important symbolic meanings that bear on individual and social well-being. Analyses that attempt to statistically separate race and class have been criticized for failing to recognize that such factors are inextricably bound. As one author writes, "African Americans do not just happen to be over-represented in low socioeconomic strata; rather, a higher proportion of African Americans than U.S. whites are represented in low socioeconomic classification because of the continuing significance of what it means to be black in U.S. society."[40] In other words, the category of race is socially meaningful in the United States because of the connection between racism and inequality. Many posit that blacks' socioeconomic disadvantage can be properly understood only as a *result* of racial discrimination and that attempts to sort out race and class will generally fall short.

Supporting such arguments of race's continued significance is evidence suggesting that racism in day-to-day life contributes to differences in health. Darker skin color appears to be an important determinant of exposure to racial discrimination and unequal access to resources,[41] and studies have found that darker skin color is associated with higher levels of hypertension for middle- and upper-class blacks.[42] In the context of American race dynamics, dark skin is associated with lower social status, and the incongruity between dark skin color and high socioeconomic status may expose individuals with such characteristics to more striking cases of discrimination. Discrimination, in turn, may increase stress, ultimately elevating one's risk of hypertension.[43]

Sherman James's hypothesis of "John Henryism" is another good example of how discrimination and racial symbolism may affect health.[44] Researchers generally find that hypertension is inversely related to socioeconomic status, so that as one's education, income, and occupational prestige decrease, the risk of hypertension increases.[45] However, on the individual level, the risk of hypertension also appears to be particularly high for individuals who demonstrate "high effort" in coping with difficult psychosocial stressors—that is, actively working at trying to eliminate stressors.[46] James, drawing on the symbolism of John Henry—the legendary "steel-driving man" of the 1870s—suggests that the high risk of hypertension among African Americans can be attributed to interactions between these two risk factors and the culture of race in the United States. According to James, a legacy of slavery, combined with traditional American values of self-reliance and hard work, makes African Americans more likely not only to encounter stressors but also to take a "John Henry–like" approach to them (that is, "to engage in prolonged, high effort coping with difficult psychosocial environmental stressors").[47] Here race is not only a socioeconomic category but also a symbol that affects how people interact with one another.

Variation in the way that age affects low birth weight offers another good example of how discrimination may be linked to health. Studies have found that among blacks, but not among whites, maternal age above 15 is associated with a higher risk of low birth weight. Arline Geronimus has suggested that this association may be the result of a weathering effect of social inequality on black women. That is, as time elapses, the effects of racial inequality may accumulate physically within black women's bodies. Black women have weathered the inequality that they face for longer than their younger counterparts, and thus, according to this logic, their pregnancies are at a higher risk of low-birth-weight delivery.[48] The exact mechanisms of this hypothesis remain unclear. Increased exposure to environmental toxins may place black women at a greater risk, or cumulative stressors resulting from discrimination in day-to-day interactions may be to blame for race differences in the effects of age on birth weight. In either case, however, this argument suggests that it is the discrimination characterizing race that is central to the effects of race on health.

Racial discrimination in the United States can also be understood as a question of power differentials. In the mid-1980s John McKnight suggested that traditional public health measures were inherently flawed because they ignored the question of empowerment. The groups with the least power are generally the least healthy, and McKnight suggested that such power differentials lie at the heart of health patterns.[49] Thomas LaVeist, testing this claim, compared different metropolitan areas and found that black postneonatal mortality rates were lower in cities where African Americans had higher levels of political power, while white postneonatal mortality rates were unaffected by such a factor.[50] In this analysis, LaVeist ruled out a purely material explanation suggesting that black political empowerment improves infant health simply because black elected officials allocate resources to benefit African Americans. Rather, LaVeist found that community organizing was the salient factor, not only because it improved the material conditions of African Americans but also because it facilitated greater black political power. Such a finding suggests that economic resources are not (as class-based explanations of race emphasize) enough by themselves; political resources matter too.

While this argument presents an interesting connection between race and health, we again face problems of causation—in this case, particularly spuriousness. Politically empowered communities may differ from unempowered communities in multiple health-related ways that LaVeist does not account for. For example, recent evidence suggests that several alternative neighborhood characteristics, such as levels of social support and of violent crime, are connected to infant health.[51] Broad social networks or low levels of crime may themselves relate to community empowerment and may promote infant health, while political mobilization may have no causal role at all.

Beyond Class: The Effects of Culture on Low Birth Weight

Evidence from Mexican American births have led several authors to suggest that culture and lifestyle are the key forces driving race differences in health. Several studies have shown that Mexican American

women recently arrived in the United States give birth to full-term nor-
mal-weight babies at the same rate as whites despite their significantly
disadvantaged economic position and their minority status.[52] However,
the longer a mother has resided in the United States and the more accul-
turated she has become to American life, the higher the risk of preterm delivery and low birth weight.[53] Based on this evidence, many
researchers have concluded that, although the women just arriving
from Mexico are no better off economically than those who have been
here for some time (in fact they are likely to be worse off), they benefit
from a cultural shield of sorts. That is, their traditional diets and family
living arrangements are better suited for the low-income conditions that
Mexicans and Mexican Americans have traditionally endured. However, the transformation of these immigrants' lives into those of poor
Americans brings a worse diet, greater family instability, and higher
rates of substance abuse. Thus, a loss of Mexican cultural attributes
may explain an increased incidence of low birth weight. Welcome to
America.

However, such foreigner birth benefits have been found in other immigrant groups, such as West African–born and Caribbean-born women,
which raises questions about the validity of a specifically Mexican cultural explanation.[54] Such similar findings among these different groups
may imply, of course, that all these women share protective cultural
characteristics. However, the findings may also imply that there is something about migration itself that explains health benefits. Migration is
generally selective on socioeconomic and demographic characteristics—
meaning that people with particular economic or demographic characteristics are more likely to migrate than those without such characteristics.[55] However, migration may also be selective on traits that are not
so easily measured, such as general health status or motivation to succeed.[56] Therefore, it may be the case that women who are generally
better off are more likely to migrate to the United States, so that their
impressive birth outcomes are actually a result of their beneficial individual characteristics rather than their group culture. A recent study by
Nancy Landale and her colleagues investigates this hypothesis of selective migration by comparing Puerto Rican women who did and did
not migrate from Puerto Rico to the mainland United States. These
researchers found much better birth outcomes among recent, nonassim-
ilated Puerto Rican migrants as compared to women who remained
in Puerto Rico, suggesting that selective migration contributed to the
foreigner birth advantage found in previous research.[57] Presumably,

all women raised in Puerto Rico enjoy the same cultural advantages. So if culture was what really mattered, there would be no difference between women who recently migrated and women who did not. Evidence of such differences in this study, therefore, suggests that cultural benefits alone cannot explain the health of foreign-born women. These results seem to suggest, rather, that Puerto Rican women who are advantaged in some way are more likely to relocate and their positive birth outcomes reflect this advantage. In this case, the less positive birth outcomes that emerge after women have resided in the United States for a time could be due to the lesser access immigrants have to the U.S. health care system,[58] or perhaps to higher rates of stress or isolation found in the U.S. context as compared to the homeland context.

As evidence demonstrates, class is a crucial component of racial variation in birth outcomes, and more refined measures of class may demonstrate its even greater importance. However, the continued relationship between race and other factors, such as discrimination or cultural differences, also challenges efforts to explain race entirely in terms of class. Such mixed findings remind us that relying too heavily on any single theoretical perspective may impair a comprehensive understanding of race and health. We should again note that statistically "controlling for" race and/or class allows us to consider only direct effects. Separating out the indirect effects of race and class proves quite difficult since these factors can be tightly intertwined—both empirically and conceptually.

Consider, for instance, variations in the etiologies of low birth weight by race. As we discussed in chapter 1, low birth weight may result from either of two conditions—a preterm delivery or intrauterine growth retardation (IUGR). That is, a baby may be born small because it was born early or because it did not grow at a normal rate. Race differences in these two causes of low birth weight are quite significant. Black-white differences in the propensity for preterm birth are approximately twice as large as those differences in IUGR.[59] How does this disparity relate to socioeconomic factors? The answer is somewhat ambiguous. Cases of low birth weight resulting from preterm delivery appear to be significantly less sensitive to immediate socioeconomic conditions than those cases resulting from IUGR.[60] Indeed, Jeffrey Kallan found that, while IUGR is quite sensitive to immediate socioeconomic and demographic conditions, such as marital status, preterm delivery is far more sensitive to biological conditions, like hypertension or pelvic infections.[61]

Given the large role of preterm deliveries in the race gap in low birth weight, these findings may lead us to assume that race differences in rates of low birth weight result more from biological conditions than from socioeconomic conditions. But this assumption would overlook evidence suggesting that the health conditions associated with preterm delivery may at least partially result from the cumulative effects of low socioeconomic status. Kallan, for instance, documents that low education levels—which may reflect a childhood and/or young adulthood spent in poverty—are associated with elevated risks for the health complications associated with preterm delivery (namely, hypertension and pelvic infections).[62] Thus, while race differences in the specific causes of low birth weight (preterm delivery versus IUGR) may initially seem to suggest nonsocioeconomic—even biological—causes behind the race gap in rates of low birth weight, further investigation reveals that socioeconomic status plays at least some indirect role in the biological factors that underlie these etiological differences.

BIOLOGICAL AND GENETIC EXPLANATIONS

In stark contrast to the above discussion of race and health stand biological explanations of race that emphasize the importance of different genetic profiles in accounting for black-white health disparities. There is evidence that the incidence of some diseases is linked to genetic differences between groups—the greater propensity of African Americans to suffer from sickle-cell anemia or for Ashkenazi Jews to be afflicted with Tay-Sachs syndrome are two such examples.[63] However, other scholars have argued that even discussing genetics and race is inherently racist, and it has been estimated that only 2 percent of blacks' excess mortality can be attributed to genes.[64] In the nature-nurture debate, race occupies a particularly controversial space. As we mentioned before, the social sciences were partly a response to very dubious linkages drawn in the nineteenth century between genetics and inequality—and race was a favored topic of this work. Correctly fearing a return to such so-called science, many researchers (both biologists and social scientists) have avoided considering genetic explanations of racial differences in health. Because of the practical and political implications, such work can be quite complicated. When considering genetics and race, as in the following analysis, we must pay close attention to the intimate connections between genes and environment and—in attempting to avoid a reductionist approach—must keep in mind that a genetic difference does not necessarily imply a purely biological force or a "predetermined" disparity.

While there is no direct evidence of a racially based gene for birth weight, some evidence does suggest biological and/or genetic explanations for racial differences in low birth weight. One of the most noted points in biological explanations of black-white differences in low birth weight is the higher rate of neonatal survival exhibited by African American low-birth-weight babies compared to their white counterparts. Given two babies born at equally low weights, the African American baby has a better chance of surviving through the neonatal period than the white baby. (However, the increased African American risk of being born low birth weight in the first place is greater than the decreased risk of neonatal mortality from low birth weight complications, so that the infant mortality rate for blacks remains twice that for whites.)

Social explanations for this survival benefit are rather hard to imagine. After all, it is difficult to believe that social disadvantage can simultaneously lead to poorer birth outcomes *and* better chances of survival given these poor outcomes. This inconsistency has lead some authors to take an alternative approach, suggesting that infants of different races may "naturally" come in different sizes due to genetic variations between the two populations. Behind this hypothesis is the assumption that, if differences in birth weight are due to a natural genetic tendency, low birth weight may have different meanings for African American and white babies. If black babies are "naturally" smaller than white babies, low birth weight for a black baby may not indicate the same level of physiological immaturity, and hence health risk, that it does for a white baby.

Gestation-specific birth weights across whole birth weight spectrums do indeed seem to point to "natural" race differences, because black babies appear to be smaller than white babies regardless of term. That is, size differences between black and white babies may result from black infants being smaller than white infants at all gestational ages.[65] Different development patterns may also point to genetic or biological differences in African American and white birth weights. Studies have found that black fetuses develop more rapidly in the first 36 weeks of gestation than do white fetuses, so that at earlier gestational ages black babies may be more physiologically mature than white babies.[66] The important implication of such a finding is that a lower birth weight or a premature birth for an African American baby may be the result not of the mother's poor health or social conditions, but rather of a "natural" tendency toward smaller babies.

Studies of mixed-race infants further support arguments for specifically genetic differences between blacks and whites. Mixed-race infants, regardless of socioeconomic status, are generally born at weights in between infants with two white parents and those with two black parents.[67] Further, the incidence of low birth weight among infants who have one black parent and one white parent (relative to those who have two white parents) is twice as large when the father is black as when the mother is black.[68] These findings suggest that each parent may contribute race-specific genes to the baby's birth weight status. This role of the father's race in determining low birth weight status is noteworthy also because the father, as a contributor of genes who does not carry the fetus, is more likely to influence fetal development through genetic characteristics than uterine ones. These different risk profiles, however, could result from the different sociodemographic profiles of white mother–black father and black mother–white father couples.

Indeed, opposing these genetic and biological explanations is a fair amount of alternative evidence. A study of low birth weight in the Czech Republic, an ethnically homogeneous country with nearly universal health coverage, found that babies of less educated single women display the same weight-specific neonatal survival advantage found among black infants in the United States.[69] Within an ethnically homogeneous population such variation could not possibly be attributed to racially based population genetics or ethnic biological variation; therefore, the many genetic and biological arguments based on survival rates may be incorrect. A study by Richard David and James Collins examining West African–born black women's birth outcomes similarly challenges specifically genetic explanations of race differences in low birth weight. These authors, hypothesizing that African American infants' smaller size may be related to their West African heritage, suggest that West African–born women—with "purely" West African genetic heritage—should give birth to infants smaller than African American women—who are assumed to have only three-quarters of their genetic makeup from West Africa. Findings from this study show, however, that West African–born women on average give birth to babies who are larger than those of African American women, contrary to the authors' hypothesis.[70]

Going beyond these particular studies, several scholars have criticized genetic arguments as scientifically untenable and socially unacceptable. Many scholars have suggested that genetic explanations of race in the United States are, in general, implausible because the category of African American is so diverse as to be genetically meaningless.[71] For instance, Richard Cooper points out that classification based on skin color is really quite arbitrary because members of a racial group are likely to share relatively few characteristics beyond skin color. As Cooper writes, "Although two groups may be similar in skin color, they differ in other important features, such as height, blood type or facial features. To classify on the basis of skin color arbitrarily assigns primary importance to that characteristic and forces all others to be ignored."[72] In other words, while skin color is of grave importance in social categorization, biological similarities based on skin color are limited.

Such shaky biological evidence, combined with black-white patterns of health care receipt and socioeconomic differentiation, have led some to suggest that discussing race and genetics is inherently racist. Jacqueline Stevens points out that racism stems from views about innate differences, and medical research now emphasizing such innate differences with genetic research may be hardening the very theoretical basis of racism.[73] In other words, genetic research may widen current health differentials by fostering the very attitudes associated with residential, occupational, and wealth segregation.

A related critique of genetic approaches is offered by Troy Duster in his book *Back Door to Eugenics*.[74] Duster criticizes public health policies that focus on genetic screenings for diseases such as sickle-cell anemia and Tay-Sachs syndrome, arguing that such seemingly objective scientific approaches are in fact strongly influenced by social power dynamics. It is no coincidence, Duster argues, that genetically "at risk" populations overlap with social categories of race, ethnicity, and sex. Further, Duster suggests that, when such social-genetic categories influence public health policy, eugenic tendencies develop. Referring specifically to prenatal screenings, Duster writes: "This kind of screen heavily implies that if one finds what one is looking for, then termination of the pregnancy is high on the list of potential intervention strategies. . . . The new technologies move large, impersonal forces almost inexorably to 'screen' against such 'outcomes' in 'cost-effective' terms."[75] Given the complicated social context in which research on race and health is carried out, in addition to the troubled legacy of research on race and genetics, considering race and biology can be problematic. Indeed, given race relations in the United States, we often cannot be sure that even the most well-intentioned research on race and health is "objective" or benign. Yet, when blacks face greater than twice the risk as whites of low birth weight, it can be difficult—and perhaps even harmful—to ignore race as a risk factor in health.

Given the evidence that seems to pile up against completely social or completely biological/genetic explanations of race and health, it is helpful to remember that society and biology are not as polarized as is often assumed. An individual's genetic makeup is the result of a long process of reproduction that is governed by social norms and patterns. Mating is not random. People tend to have children with people who are similar to them, and one of the starkest divisions in these patterns of mating is race. African Americans are far more likely to have a child with another African American than with a white person, and white people are far more likely to have a child with another white person than with an African American. Such a pattern creates a stratified reproduction process and, thus, may place blacks or whites at disproportionate risk for certain genetically linked health conditions. Such a connection between the social and the possible genetic implications of race does not mean, however, that race is a genetic fact. Rather, race is a social category that has certain biological implications. If society were stratified based on some other principle, say hair color, over time people with particular hair colors might conceivably begin to face a disproportionate risk of certain genetic compositions. This of course does not mean that hair color itself places people at a genetic advantage or disadvantage but rather that the social meaning of hair color places people in such a position.

RESEARCH QUESTIONS AND DATA

In this chapter we address several questions about the roles of nature and nurture in African American and white rates of low birth weight. First, we consider to what extent low birth weight is heritable. Does parental low birth weight represent a biological propensity toward filial low birth weight or the reproduction of social conditions across generations? Second, we consider whether a historical legacy of low birth weight accounts for the higher propensity of African Americans to be born low birth weight. That is, is a historical biological propensity for low birth weight more important for blacks than whites, and if so, can biology explain blacks' elevated rates of low birth weight? Coupling such biological factors with social factors in the following analysis will also allow us to address the larger question of whether a family history of low birth weight implies a family with "unfortunate" genes or a family with a disadvantaged environment.

There is notable variation in birth weight across several racial and ethnic groups in the United States besides blacks and whites (i.e., Latinos, Native Americans, and Asians).[76] However, we choose not to examine these groups and to classify our Panel Study of Income Dynamics (PSID) sample into black and nonblack because the greatest discrepancies in birth weight in the U.S. population are between blacks and other groups. Thus, from here on, comparisons within our sample are between blacks and nonblacks, as opposed to blacks and whites. Due to the profound social significance of race, we incorporate this racial categorization into our statistical analyses.

STATISTICAL APPROACH: ESTIMATING
HERITABILITY USING THREE GENERATIONS

Our strategy is to examine the effects of parents' birth weights and socioeconomic statuses on the likelihood of a low birth weight birth. First, we examine how parents' social and biological characteristics might explain racial differences in birth weight, factoring out other variables that are associated with birth weight (mother's age, marital status, and education; infant's sex and firstborn status). Next, we examine whether the importance of parents' social and biological characteristics vary by race, factoring out the other important variables listed above. If, after we have factored out socioeconomic and other relevant differences, the residual effect of race is eliminated by addressing parents' birth weights, medical history differences may possibly—but not definitively—explain the race effect not explained by class. In addition, if the father's birth weight status affects the infant's, regardless of the mother's, we may come closer to concluding that genetics plays a role, since, as discussed above, the father's contribution is more likely to be genetic than the mother's.

In some of the models in this chapter we employ standard statistical techniques that compare one family to a random set of other families. However, as we discussed before, such comparisons can potentially be confounded by the presence of additional, unobserved factors causing different families' tendencies toward low birth weight. For instance, in these models aspects of the home environment or maternal health characteristics that we do not have information on may give us spurious results. To deal with such a problem of unobserved variables we repeat all of our analyses using family fixed-effects models—that is, comparing individuals in the same extended family. Specifically, in these analyses we compare cousins who have the same maternal grandparents.

When comparing cousins in this analysis, we are basically holding constant the contributions that maternal grandparents may make to future biological, environmental, and behavioral conditions and are thereby eliminating some of the variance between families that may bias our cross-family comparisons (while also maintaining variance among parents that would be lost in sibling comparisons, for example). The attention to maternal grandparents in this analysis is quite important because ignoring variation in earlier generations may make it quite difficult to understand the true mechanisms behind low birth weight. Imagine, for example, a family in which the grandmother and the mother smoked the mother and the grandchild were born low birth weight. In this case, where both biological and environmental/behavioral conditions are being passed along generations, how might causation be working? On one hand, the grandmother's smoking could cause her daughter to be born of low birth weight and to smoke later in life; the daughter's smoking could then lead to the low birth weight status of the grandchild. On the other hand, there could be no causal connection between smoking and low birth weight in this family. In that case, the grandmother's smoking would lead to the mother's smoking, but it would be the grandmother's birth weight status that led to the mother's birth weight status, and the mother's birth weight status that led to the grandchild's birth weight status. In this case, filial birth weight is caused by biological inheritance, and intergenerational smoking patters are an unrelated phenomenon.

Biological and behavioral/environmental variation in earlier generations can clearly make it difficult to sort out the causal factors behind low birth weight—biological and behavioral/environmental causation appeared equally feasible in this scenario. Using within-family comparisons, however, we will be able to hold constant such unobserved differences. Given that cousin comparisons essentially factor out a portion of unobserved environmental and genetic variation, the intergenerational differences in birth weight we find (after controlling for socioeconomic factors) are probably a relatively pure biological effect. As shown in Figure 2.1, in comparing the birth weights of two maternal cousins, we are really comparing the pregnancies of two sisters. Since these two sisters were born to the same parents and likely grew up in the same household, a fair amount of unaccounted-for variation has been

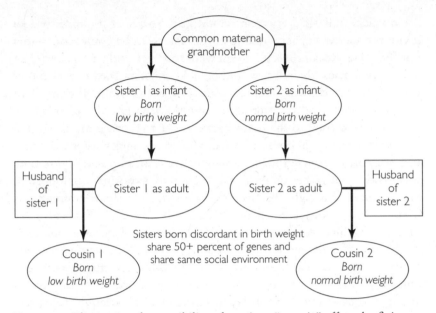

Figure 2.1. Eliminating the possibility of spurious "genetic" effects by fixing grandparents

eliminated. This means that discordant birth weights replicated across two generations have arisen despite relatively low levels of general variance and, therefore, may represent a biological cause of low birth weight.

We can be so confident about the meanings of our results, precisely because cousin comparisons place strict limitations on *how* unobserved variance may bias those results. Let us consider, for instance, the possibility of bias resulting from environmental factors—specifically, exposure to toxins. Toxins may seem a relatively likely source of bias for these models since some toxins have direct intergenerational effects (harming the reproductive capacity of not only the mother but also her baby) and intergenerational patterns of birth weight discordance are what concerns us. However, examining the requirements of cousin comparisons more closely, we see that even this intergenerational source of bias is probably not common or systematic enough to affect our results. Let us consider two toxins that are known to have negative effects on reproductive capacity across generations—lead and diethyl-stilbestrol (also know as DES, a synthetic estrogen drug that was given to pregnant women between 1938 and 1971 and that had adverse health effects).[77] In order for one of these toxins to bias our estimates of a biological, inherited effect, it would have to affect the birth weight and reproductive capacity of one of the sisters in the comparison—but not the other. Recall that, if a toxin were to affect both sisters and their later pregnancies, the effect would be held constant (i.e., canceled out) because we are drawing comparisons only within familial pairs. This constraint, practically speaking, means that the grandmother would have to be exposed to the toxin between her two pregnancies, so that the older sister would not be affected while the younger sister would be. It is possible of course for the grandmother to be exposed *before* both pregnancies but rather unlikely that such early exposure would lead to discordant birth weights between the two sisters. It is hard to imagine a toxin that is strong enough to affect the birth weight (and also the future reproductive capacity) of the first sister but lacks the long-term implications for the mother's reproductive system that would affect her second pregnancy. Thus, for a toxin, or any other potential bias, to significantly alter our results it must produce discordant birth weights among siblings—that is, the bias must take place between the two pregnancies—and it must be replicated across generations.

If we consider the practicalities of potential sources of bias, we see that our model's constraints significantly limit the sources' possible effects. For example, while DES easily satisfies the requirement of intergenerational replication, it is unlikely that this drug was prescribed in between two pregnancies on so regular a basis that our randomly drawn sample would be significantly affected. In this case, the constraints imposed by the cousin comparison mean that it is simply unlikely that this source of bias, in this specific pattern, is widespread enough to alter our results—particularly since most babies in our sample were born after its use was discontinued in 1971. In the case of lead, bias becomes practically impossible. For lead to have deleterious effects on health and reproductive capacity, exposure usually has to take place early in an individual's childhood—long before puberty or any pregnancy.[78] This practical necessity virtually eliminates the possibility that lead poisoning could take place between two pregnancies, affecting one but not the other.

Among behavioral sources of variation, likely bias is even harder to find. With behavioral sources of bias (and many other environmental sources as well) we cannot take intergenerational replication for granted as we did with DES and lead. This means we must be able to find a behavior that affects one pregnancy but not the other and that is replicated across generations. While it is certainly possible that a mother would, say, smoke during only one pregnancy and the low birth weight daughter from this pregnancy would smoke during her pregnancy (while her normal-birth-weight sister remained smoke free while pregnant), it is again unlikely that this specific pattern would occur on such a wide scale as to significantly bias our randomly drawn sample. The confines placed on behavioral and environmental patterns by cousin fixed-effects models make it rather difficult to identify serious potential sources of bias.

While cousin comparisons make it quite likely that we will uncover true, unbiased genetic effects in this analysis, there are still further ways to boost confidence in our results. As mentioned above, environmental or behavioral variation would likely have to take place between the grandmother's two pregnancies. This means that, if environmental and behavioral bias is a serious concern, we should see more second children born low birth weight than first children.[79] However, when testing for this potential, we do not find such a pattern—birth order–birth weight interactions are statistically insignificant. We are also more likely to find behavioral and/or environmental variation among low-income groups than high-income groups. Given socioeconomic patterns, a low-income grandmother is more likely to have smoked or been exposed to toxins than a high-income grandmother. This implies that, if differences between the sisters' birth weights are greater in the lower-income portion of our sample than in the higher-income portion, we would have reason to be concerned about unobserved variance. However, our results show no such variation across income categories. Rather, after splitting our sample based on high and low income, we find levels of birth weight discordance to be close to uniform across socioeconomic status. That is, none of our tests gives us reason to believe that there is significant behavioral or environmental bias at work in these estimates.

THE INHERITANCE OF LOW BIRTH WEIGHT

Our analysis begins with a simple model that compares the risk of low birth weight across race and proceeds to factor out other important characteristics in an attempt to account for racial differences. In Figure 2.2, the first bar (simply contrasting black and white likelihood of low birth weight) shows that blacks are much—109 percent—more likely than nonblacks to be born below 2,500 grams. (Please refer to appendix A for details regarding the calculation of changes in probability.)

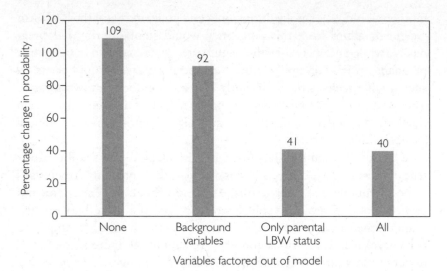

Figure 2.2. The impact of race on filial low birth weight (LBW): the percentage increase, as compared to nonblacks, in the probability of an LBW birth associated with African Americans, using between-family models. See appendix B, Table 2.1, for descriptive statistics related to these variables; Table 2.3 (models A, C, D, and E, respectively) for regression coefficients associated with this analysis.

The second bar in Figure 2.2 shows that, after factoring out the respondent's characteristics (i.e., sex and firstborn status) and the socioeconomic variables (i.e., income-to-needs ratio and mother's education, marital status, and age), the effect of race is significantly reduced. In light of all these additional variables, African Americans are now 92 percent more likely than their non–African American counterparts to be born of low birth weight. Comparing the first and second bars of the graph, we find that respondents' characteristics and this particular set of socioeconomic variables accounted for approximately 17 percentage points of the previous 109 percent risk difference found when comparing across race without additional controls.

The third bar in Figure 2.2 compares black and nonblack likelihood of low birth weight when only parental low-birth-weight status is factored out. Addressing parents' biological legacies in such a manner reduces the effect of race so that now blacks are only 41 percent more likely to be born low birth weight. Comparing this bar to the second, which factored out respondent characteristics and socioeconomic variables, we note that parents' birth-weight status has a much stronger effect on race differences than respondents' characteristics and socioeco-

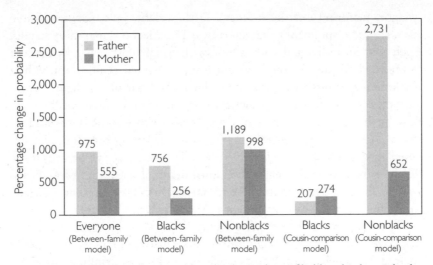

Figure 2.3. The impact of parental low birth weight on filial low birth weight, by race: the percentage increase in the probability of low birth weight (LBW) associated with having an LBW parent, using between-family and cousin-comparison models. See appendix B, Table 2.1, for descriptive statistics related to these variables; Table 2.4 (both columns) for regression coefficients for logistic models; Table 2.5 for regression coefficients associated with fixed-effects models.

nomic variables combined. This implies that it is the previous generation's health status (and whatever it may be acting as proxy for)—more than the current social conditions—that explains the lion's share of race differences in the current generation's birth outcomes. This finding implies that the studies outlined above that find current social conditions to be of great importance may reflect, at least in part, an association between health and social conditions that spans generations. Evidence of the "effects" of current social conditions may be inflated, partially reflecting the noncausal association between social conditions and health; the health status of earlier generations—not accounted for in these studies—may be playing the causal role. The last bar in Figure 2.2 shows the residual effect of race that remains even after factoring out the respondents' characteristics, socioeconomic variables, and parental birth weight. Even taking account of all these additional characteristics, race still has an effect, albeit reduced, on low birth weight.

Trying to better understand the effect of parental low birth weight, we break down the parental birth weight effects into maternal and paternal effects in Figure 2.3. The first bar in this figure represents the risk of low birth weight for an individual whose father was low birth weight, factoring out the mother's birth weight, race, socioeconomic factors, and respondent's characteristics. The effect is remarkably strong, such that an individual with a low-birth-weight father is 975 percent more likely to be low birth weight him- or herself than an individual without a low-birth-weight father. The second bar in this figure represents the risk of low birth weight for an individual whose mother was low birth weight, regardless of the father's birth weight status and all the above variables. This effect is not quite as strong but still quite sizable; an individual with a low-birth-weight mother is 555 percent more likely to be low birth weight than an individual with a non-low-birth-weight mother. These maternal and paternal effects represent a unique contribution made by each parent to the baby's birth weight.

The uniqueness of these effects may imply that they are more likely to be genetic, since social conditions (like income or race) are usually shared. Even behavioral factors (such as smoking or drinking) are more often shared and thus would not be picked up in these variables, which are unique to each parent. How shared are the genetic propensities to be born of low birth weight? That would depend on the level of assortative mating on the criteria of low birth weight status. In other words, do individuals who are low birth weight tend to marry others who are low birth weight? To the extent that they do (the correlation among parents' birth weight statuses in our sample is rather low, at .223), our estimates are biased downward.

We are not yet working here with cousin fixed-effects models, so it is a bit unclear why the maternal effect is somewhat weaker than the paternal effect. As we discussed above, the effects of paternal low-birth-weight status are more likely to represent a genetic effect, since the father cannot affect the fetus via the uterine environment in the same direct way the mother can. This greater paternal effect may therefore imply that genetics matter more for birth weight status than the prenatal environment does. However, we ought to be cautious in accepting such a limited role for the prenatal environment, given all the evidence suggesting the importance of the mother's behavior while pregnant.

We also tested for sex linkage in the transmission of low birth weight. Only fathers contribute the Y chromosome to sons, so if paternal low birth weight status has a stronger effect on sons' birth weight status than on daughters', the Y chromosome—that is, genetic transmission—would be at work in this association. When comparing paternal effects across sons and daughters, however, we do not find such a difference. This result, while not supporting a genetic explanation, also does not rule out a genetic explanation, since transmission could still be taking place through other chromosomes that are not sex specific.

The larger paternal effect could also be the result of some sort of bias, such as that associated with recall. Information on fathers' birth weight status is often not as readily available as that on mothers' (frequently because the father is not present). We can therefore imagine that if a mother being interviewed about her child's birth weight status is queried about the father's birth weight status and the information is not immediately available, she may be more likely to assume he was low birth weight in order to make sense of her child's low birth weight. We do not, however, have any information to document such a scenario, and it is questionable that such recall bias would take place on a large enough scale to render differences of this size between paternal and maternal effects.

To test whether the inheritance of low birth weight varies by race, we compare the strength of each maternal and paternal effect for blacks and nonblacks in the next two pairs of bars in Figure 2.3. Here we note that the effects of parental low birth weight vary significantly by race. The effect of mother's low birth weight is significantly smaller for African Americans than for non–African Americans: having a low-birth-weight mother increases the probability that a black baby will be born low birth weight by 256 percent. In contrast, a low-birth-weight mother increases the risk of low birth weight for a nonblack baby by 998 percent. Black-nonblack differences in paternal effect are not statistically significant. This lesser effect of maternal low birth weight among blacks as compared to nonblacks (and the nonsignificant differences in paternal effects) leads us to reject the possibility that there is a higher degree of biological inheritance (i.e., a greater genetic component) of low birth weight within the African American community than within other groups. These findings do not imply, however, that there is *no* genetic inheritance of birth weight within the African American community, but rather that parental birth weight status is a weaker predictor among African Americans than among whites. We will explore possible reasons for this later in this chapter.

THE INHERITANCE OF LOW BIRTH WEIGHT WITHIN FAMILIES

In order to further test whether we are witnessing biological effects in these coefficients for parental low birth weight, we performed the above analysis again, but this time by comparing maternal cousins. Even within this stricter model, shown in the last two pairs of bars of Figure 2.3, maternal and paternal low birth weights have an important impact on filial low birth weight that continues to vary by race. In this fixed-effects framework, the effect of father's low birth weight is significantly smaller for African Americans than for non–African Americans. Having a low-birth-weight father increases the probability that a black baby will be born low birth weight, by 207 percent, whereas a low-birth-weight father increases the risk of low birth weight by 2,731 percent for a nonblack baby. Race differences in maternal effects are rather small in this framework. Because we are working with family fixed-effects models now, the likelihood that the maternal and paternal effects represent biological transmission is reversed. In the cross-family models discussed above, we assumed the paternal effect was more likely biological given that the father does not carry the fetus. In these cousin comparisons, we have eliminated large amounts of variation from the mother's side, so it now becomes more likely that the mother's effect is biological in nature. These results—across both race categories— therefore suggest a combination of biological and nonbiological inheritance. That is, since the maternal grandparents are factored out in this model but the paternal grandparent effects may remain, the difference between the maternal and paternal effects tells us that a certain amount of the inheritance (part of the paternal effect) may not be biological but a sizable amount (the maternal effect) may be.

When we compare across race using both traditional and between-family models, we again find that the inheritance patterns are stronger for nonblacks than blacks. Both maternal and paternal low birth weight appear to have stronger effects for nonblacks than for blacks. However, with our fixed-effects models the difference in the effect of maternal low birth weight is not statistically significant, while the difference in paternal low birth weight is. This suggests that the differences in inheritance are perhaps found in the persistence of "social" factors rather than biological ones, especially given the reverse pattern in the non-fixed-effects results—namely, the racial difference in the effect of mothers (the more environmentally affected parent in this case) being more pronounced.

Let us investigate the meaning of these race differences in inheritance (found in both our between- and within-family models) with a mental experiment. Let us imagine a sample of 100 African American pregnancies and 100 non–African American pregnancies. Further, let us assume that 10 percent of this entire population has a genetic tendency toward low birth weight, regardless of race. This means that, if social factors were held constant across these racial groups, there would be ten low-birth-weight births in the black population and ten such births in the nonblack population. But because the African American population is likely facing greater environmental and social risk than the non–African American population, we find instead of such straightforward results, say, 20 low-birth-weight (LBW) births in our African American population and ten LBW births in the non–African American population. This would imply that, among the black population, the ten pregnancies with genetic tendencies resulted in LBW births, but then an additional ten pregnancies resulted in LBW births because of social risk factors. Meanwhile, among our non–African American population, only the ten pregnancies with genetic tendencies resulted in LBW births. (We are assuming there were no LBW births resulting from social factors in this half of our sample.) While the same number of births were low birth weight because of genetic tendencies in both the African American and non–African American populations, the proportion of low-birth-weight births that were the result of genetic tendencies is still lower among the African Americans than among the non–African Americans. While 100 percent of the LBW births in our non–African American population can be attributed to genetics, only 50 percent of the LBW births in our African American population can be so attributed. It is likely a difference such as this—a difference in the proportion of low birth weight births that can be attributed to genetics—that is responsible for the weaker African American inheritance we find in both our between-family and within-family models. This situation, in which the effect of inheritance is "diluted" because of higher social risk, is also supported by the last bar in Figure 2.3, which shows that African Americans still face a 40 percent higher risk of a low birth weight birth, even after factoring out background characteristics, socioeconomic characteristics, and parental low birth weight.

African Americans seem to face additional risk factors, independent of inheritance, that likely make the effect of inheritance weaker. This socially based interpretation is bolstered by the fact that, when we examine cross-family models, where the father's contribution is more likely to be genetic and less likely to be environmental, it is the mother's effects that vary by race. But when we deploy maternal-grandmother fixed-effects models so that the impact of father's birth weight is more likely to be acting as proxy for social effects, then it is the fathers who demonstrate a significant racial difference in their impact, while mothers—whose birth weight effects in this case may be more purely genetic since they are sisters who shared the same family conditions growing up—demonstrate a lesser race difference.

In light of these findings, we may reasonably conclude that there does exist a biological (possibly genetic) component to the intergenerational transmission of low birth weight and that this inheritance does contribute to race differences in the risk of low birth weight. However, the degree and form of social and biological heritability may vary by race. Our findings also point to the importance of fathers in birth weight, regardless of the degree of inheritance among African Americans and non–African Americans. Few have studied paternal factors, and thus future researchers would do well to consider the medical and socioeconomic histories of both parents when developing models of low birth weight risk. Uterine environment may be important, but our findings suggest it is not everything. Pregnancy presents a unique and intimate intertwining of genetics, biology, and society, and our efforts to sort out these factors suggest that they each make a unique contribution to birth weight. Consequently, makers of health policy relating to children would be wise to consider the characteristics of their mothers and fathers, as well as their grandparents'.

CHAPTER 3

What Money Can and Can't Buy

Income and Infant Health

The pound of flesh which I demand of him
Is dearly bought as mine, and I will have it.
  William Shakespeare,
  The Merchant of Venice

The diseases we grapple with have changed dramatically over the past centuries. In the 1800s, when modern medicine did not exist and housing and sanitation were poor at best, infectious diseases, such as diphtheria, measles, typhoid fever, and tuberculosis, were the main killers. Today, with modern sanitation and housing, the benefits of medical innovations, and the resulting vastly improved life expectancies, chronic conditions and degenerative diseases—such as cancer or heart disease— are the central causes of death.[1] Yet despite such profound changes in risk factors and diseases, we face essentially the same puzzle we faced hundreds of years ago—how can we explain socioeconomic differences in health?

The association between socioeconomic status and health is remarkably resilient, transcending centuries and national boundaries. Studying deaths in France in the early 1800s, Louis René Villermé found that managers, merchants, and directors could expect to live 28.2 years, while factory workers could expect to live only 17.6 years.[2] Jumping ahead 150 years or so to the 1980s, the Whitehall study similarly found starkly different life expectancies across occupational classes. Collected over a ten-year period, the Whitehall data found that age-standardized mortality rates for men ages 40 to 65 were three and a half times as high for those in lower-grade occupations as for those in higher-grade occupations.[3]

Life expectancies have improved dramatically since Villermé collected his data in the 1800s—most people alive today can expect to survive into their seventies or eighties. Yet the socioeconomic gradient in life expectancies—and health in general—has remained.

Infant health is by no means immune to these persistent class differences. As long ago as 1867, Karl Marx noted disparities in infant mortality across high- and low-income neighborhoods in England.[4] Contemporary data from the United States reflect these same sorts of disparities, with recent differences in infant mortality rates across the highest and lowest income categories as large as 300 percent.[5] Such contemporary class-based differences in infant health can even be found in countries with universal access to health care. For instance, in the Netherlands—a country with universal health care as well as an inequality index much lower than the United States'—lower socioeconomic status remains associated with elevated risks of low birth weight and infant mortality.[6] Our discussion of poverty and low birth weight thus speaks to an old question, fundamental to social epidemiology— how and why does class affect health?

At first glance, the connection between class and health may seem straightforward. For example, a simple—but incomplete—explanation is that the poor do not have enough money to stay healthy, while the rich do. But money in itself can have no real effect on health outcomes. Rather it is the meaning of money and the resources one obtains with money that may promote health. The question then becomes, what particular sorts of resources and benefits that come with more money and a higher-class position promote health? That is, what sorts of mechanisms might explain a class-health relationship? This question becomes quite puzzling when we examine the specifics. Considering first the historical evidence, we can again note the persistence of socioeconomic gradients in health across drastically different historical conditions. Given that a high income or status in the 1800s clearly secured very different resources and benefits than a high income or status does today, the resources or benefits of class position that promote health must exist across the very different conditions found throughout history. Also, even choosing just one point in time, we can complicate several simple explanations of class-health relationships by noting the wide variety of health conditions socioeconomic status influences. For instance, today, low socioeconomic status is associated with elevated risk for each of the 14 major cause-of-death categories in the International Classification of Diseases, ranging from car accidents to HIV/AIDS to cardiovascular disease.[7] This, additionally, implies that any plausible explanation of socioeconomic effects must speak to a wide variety of biological conditions and behaviors.

These complexities that we encounter when trying to explain socioeconomic factors in health have led some authors to cast a broad theoretical net, suggesting that general and fundamental aspects of class are responsible for health patterns. Some authors have suggested, for example, that class position is fundamentally tied to levels of stress that determine one's general health risk.[8] According to this argument, being at the bottom of a social hierarchy is inherently stressful, leading to worse health for those who live at that level, while being at the top is inherently less stressful, thus promoting better health. Stress levels have been linked to a wide variety of health outcomes, and data collected on nonhuman primates have suggested that social position is linked to levels of stress hormones.[9] Other authors have suggested, by contrast, that social position is consistently associated with disease because social position embodies general resources, like knowledge, money, power, and prestige, that can be use to obtain health resources in most social/ historical conditions.[10] There is evidence to support this claim. A study of the use and benefits associated with disease screens—pap smears and mammograms—found that high-status individuals are more likely to use and benefit from recently developed screening techniques.[11] Because high-status women are more likely than lower-status women to use such new technology they are ultimately less likely to die from cervical or breast cancer. Thus, as individuals in different classes are more or less able to take advantage of recently discovered and publicized health resources, we witness a relatively consistent reshaping of the mortality distribution by socioeconomic status.

While both of these general explanations are helpful in making sense of ongoing discrepancies in health, they may fail to speak to more specific empirical puzzles surrounding health and class. Such narrow questions may be just as important as larger questions, as narrow questions frequently point to the particular mechanisms that may be addressed by policy efforts. Public health policy that addresses particular risk profiles is far easier to build than policy that eliminates fundamental aspects of social hierarchy.

Among the narrower empirical debates in the literature on health are concerns over what *type* of relationship associates class with health. Several studies have found that economic resources have a stronger effect on the health of those in the lowest socioeconomic strata than for those in other strata, while a similar number of studies have found that economic resources affect the health of all people uniformly. That is, some researchers have found a nonlinear effect—an amount of money, say $500, has a stronger positive effect on the health of poorer individuals than on the health of better-off individuals—while other researchers have found a linear effect, whereby an additional $500 has the same effect on everyone. Studies documenting a nonlinear relationship generally find that additional funds make one healthier but only up to a certain point (usually about the median household income), beyond which additional funds have only a small effect on one's health.[12] James House and his colleagues, for instance, report that health gains in 1990 due to income were small for households earning more than $20,000 per year.[13] Such evidence of an income threshold is often thought to imply that access to basic necessities is the driving force behind a class-health relationship. If income really matters only for those people who are very poor, it must be impoverishment—the denial of basic resources—that explains class differences in health.

By contrast, evidence documenting a linear income effect suggests that class differences in health exist beyond the point of basic needs. For example, some studies suggest that there is a stepwise progression in the relationship between socioeconomic status and health, so that even above a certain threshold one can find rather substantial differences in health. The most impressive documentation of this relationship can be found in the Whitehall study. Comparing British civil servants who were all employed in stable white-collar jobs, researchers found that each improved grade of employment had lower levels of mortality and better health status. While the overall range in mortality between the lowest and highest grade of employment was quite large (three and a half–fold), this large difference was composed of smaller differences as the grades improved.[14] Here again we confront the problem of mechanisms. All of the members of the Whitehall study were employed in office jobs with equally low environmental risk. Even those in the lowest grades were relatively well paid compared to the general population, and since Great Britain has a single-payer universal health care system, access to health care was not at issue, either. The income differences between the groups were also so small that higher-scale workers were not likely buying a significant amount of "extra" health services.

In addition to this ambiguity about the type of relationship linking class and health, there is ambiguity as to the real meaning of class. Poor people not only have less money but also tend to behave differently than rich people—eating different foods and spending their leisure time in different ways, working different types of jobs, and using medical care in different ways than their better-off counterparts. Some authors have even suggested that the poor have different attitudes and values than wealthier people. Given all of this, we are left wondering whether class differences in health can really be attributed to economics alone. Do the poor and the wealthier differ only in terms of the money they have at their disposal, or are there differences beyond money— differences in attitudes, tastes, dispositions, even self-concepts—that may account for health disparities? Returning to our discussion of causation, we can frame this question in terms of spuriousness. Are there unobserved variables associated with both income and health that are driving the relationship between socioeconomic status and health? The answers to these questions not only point to possible mechanisms responsible for class differences in health but also have profound implications for the way we address the health-class gradient. If on one hand differences in health are the result of unequal economic resources, narrowing class differences in health would require reducing differences in economic resources. If on the other hand class differences in health are noneconomic—driven by differences in behaviors, tastes, or attitudes— policy directions become less obvious.

When considering a highly heritable biological condition, like birth weight, the many noneconomic conditions surrounding class also raise the issue of reverse causation. Since biological conditions are often associated with class, discerning which of these factors is leading to the health status and which to the economic status of the next generation can be difficult. If a poor mother passes on a propensity for low birth weight to her child and this child's low birth weight status then leads to low socioeconomic status, we have biological causation. However, if a poor mother's economic conditions lead to a low-birth-weight birth and then the child inherits the mother's low level of human capital, we have economic causation. The strong association between the noneconomic condition of poor health and the economic condition of low income makes it difficult to discern in which direction causation is running. This question also has important implications for how we address class differences in health. Economic causation implies we ought to address income differences, while biological causation implies addressing health status.

The goal of this chapter is to sort out these problems of causal directionality by isolating the biological impact of parental low birth weight and the social impact of parental income. The results that follow suggest that biological risk plays an important role in low birth weight—that is, we find that having a parent who was born low birth weight significantly increases the chances that a child will be born low birth weight. But our results also suggest that such biological transmission depends on a family's economic situation—low income, according to our results, increases the chances that parental low birth weight will translate into filial low birth weight. In the next chapter we build on these results, tracing the long-term effects of low birth weight for the infants we study in this chapter. Sorting out these various influences, we can better understand how society and biology interact over time to create a class gradient in health.

POVERTY AND LOW BIRTH WEIGHT: ACCESS TO BASIC NECESSITIES

The question of basic necessities that is frequently used to explain a non-linear relationship between class and health appears rather straightforward. If a woman does not have enough money to buy nutritious food, adequate housing, or medical services, her low income is blocking her access to *biological* necessities. Such a close connection between income and biological needs creates a very direct and intuitively appealing association between class and health, which is at least partially empirically supported. For instance, studies of severe famine in the Netherlands during World War II have found that consuming fewer than 1,000 calories per day results in dramatic reductions in pregnancy weight gain and infant birth size.[15] This association between caloric intake and health demonstrates a very clear relationship between access to resources and biological health. However, relying too heavily on such strict connections may also obscure parts of the relationship between class and health.

At the conceptual level, a discussion of deprivation generally requires us to consider income as a threshold—as a question of haves and have-nots. At the research and policy level, such a discussion requires calculating and pegging this threshold at a given level—usually the federal poverty line. The federal poverty measure attempts to draw such a line by setting a series of dollar amounts representing minimum standards of economic resources for families of various sizes. Families of a given size with incomes above the appropriate, federally defined poverty level are assumed to be able to secure adequate food, housing, and so forth, while families of equivalent size with incomes below the appropriate poverty line are assumed to be without such access. This federal threshold does indeed prove to have strong associations with infant health and mortality. For example, babies born to a mother living below the poverty line have been shown to face an increased risk of low birth weight; partially as a result of this increased risk of low birth weight, they also face a 50 percent greater risk of dying in the first year of life than a baby born to a mother living above the poverty line.[16] However, to complicate matters, poverty does not appear to have equally deleterious effects on different racial and ethnic subgroups. Rather, poverty's effects on infant health seem to vary significantly by race. Several studies have found that poverty increased the incidence of low birth weight for whites but not for blacks (although blacks have a higher risk of being born low birth weight at all socioeconomic levels).[17] In a similar vein, James Collins and his colleagues have found that for Hispanics, urban poverty is negatively associated with birth weight "only when the mother is Puerto Rican or a U.S.-born member of another subgroup."[18] Such variation in the effects of poverty on infant health can lead us to questions of conceptualization and measurement. These racial/ethnic differences may imply that a single, absolute income threshold is not accurately measuring access to resources. Even below the absolute federal poverty line, some people may be denied more than other people, and this difference in resources could have unobserved implications for health.

A fair amount of evidence does suggest that the federal poverty measure is somewhat crude. To begin with, some data suggest that the federal poverty measure is out-of-date. The federal poverty thresholds were originally created in the 1960s using measures for a minimally adequate diet as defined by the U.S. Department of Agriculture.[19] At that time, it was assumed that food usually represented about one-third of total family expenditures and that remaining funds would prove adequate to cover other basic necessities. Thus, to determine the amount that defined basic access, the money needed for an adequate diet was simply tripled and has been adjusted for inflation ever since. Such a ratio of food to other expenditures, however, is questionable given the considerable changes in the costs of living over the past three decades. A poverty line based on food costs may not adequately account for the fact that housing and job-related expenses (e.g., commuting and child care costs) have risen significantly and, hence, consume an increasingly large share of poor families' incomes.[20] Increases in the cost of health care over the past 40 years have similarly caused such expenditures to consume a larger percentage of an average household budget, from less than 5 percent in the 1950s to 6 percent in the 1980s.[21]

The existence of the so-called "near-poor" may also suggest that the poverty line is not capturing the whole picture. Families categorized as near-poor generally have incomes between 100 and 185 percent of the poverty line yet, despite their incomes, frequently have trouble making ends meet. Further, because the near-poor are generally ineligible for many government programs, they may be in even more dire straits than the officially poor—again, despite their higher incomes—when trying to obtain food, shelter, and medical care. For example, in many states Medicaid is available only to those families with incomes below 133 percent of the poverty line, leaving women and children with low incomes just above the 133 percent cutoff without access to health care.[22] Living above the formal poverty line may not necessarily provide one with access to the resources needed for healthy babies. The absolute approach of the federal measure may leave out a great deal of variation within a grey area close to but not below the poverty line.

At the same time, these problems of variation occur even among those who fall below the poverty line. Evidence suggests that poverty comes in several varieties, and the single measure that accompanies the question of basic necessities may simply be unable to capture such diversity. To begin with, there is significant variation in the duration of poverty, so that some individuals fall into poverty temporarily—often because of divorce or unemployment—while others, particularly minorities, are poor for longer periods of time with little upward mobility over the life course. There is further significant variation in the severity of poverty. In 1999, 7.1 percent of children lived in extreme poverty—meaning they lived in families with incomes below 50 percent of the poverty line (in 2001 the extreme poverty line was $7,064 for a family of three).[23] While the transitory poor and those above the extreme poverty line far outnumber the consistently poor and the extremely poor,[24] this inequality in representation is more than made up for by the implications of duration and severity. The persistently poor and the extremely poor are at significantly higher risk for many adverse health conditions than are those who are transiently or "slightly" poor. Similarly, children who experience prolonged or severe poverty show larger deficits in cognitive ability and socioemotional development than children who experience only short-term or less severe poverty.[25] When we consider poverty as a potential explanation for low-birth-weight patterns, such variation is quite problematic. Two women, one transiently poor and the other persistently poor, or one extremely poor and the other falling just below the poverty line, may be similarly categorized as living in poverty at a given point in time. However, these two women's experiences of poverty clearly vary and will likely have very different effects on their health and their babies' risks of low birth weight.

If not all forms of impoverishment are the same, then exactly which forms matter the most? That is, if poverty as a general category does not adequately capture people's access to resources, attention to more specific measures of access may be the way to go. The three resources most often seen as accounting for the relationship between low income and low birth weight are diet, housing, and prenatal care. To the degree that denial of each of these specific resources predicts the risk of low birth weight (possibly independently of poverty status), we may be able to assume that deprivation counts as a mechanism behind the poverty–low birth weight link. However, while many studies refer to the importance of diet, housing, and prenatal care, concrete evidence of their effects on infant health in industrialized nations is mixed. For instance, regarding nutrition, evidence drawn from short-lived famines has been quite convincing.[26] The Dutch famine study mentioned previously found a 300-gram decrease in mean birth weight among a cohort of babies born during and shortly after the World War II famine. A longer-term follow-up of these babies into adulthood revealed even intergenerational effects of the famine. One group of authors, for example, found an excess of perinatal deaths among the grandchildren of famine-exposed women, particularly those exposed during their third trimester.[27] However, it is not clear what the causal mechanisms would be for such a three-generation effect. Presumably the famine that caused the depression in birth weight might also have damaged the reproductive systems of those fetuses. That said, the researchers found no evidence of adverse consequences of the famine on the female offspring's fertility as measured by age at menarche and the proportion having no children. Furthermore, the researchers did not examine the children of males who were in utero at the time of the famine. Men would have made a good counterexample since they do not carry the next generation in utero and thus any damage done to their reproductive system should have less of an effect on the subsequent generation's perinatal health. So we are left with a bit of a mystery.

In a contemporary U.S. context, results from nutritional studies yield far weaker results. Studies of diet in the United States have found that, while poverty increases reported difficulty in affording food, quality of diet itself does not affect birth weight.[28] Studies examining improved nutrition obtained through participation in the Supplemental Food Program for Women, Infants and Children (WIC) have revealed somewhat larger effects. WIC benefits have been found to reduce low-birth-weight rates by up to 25 percent and very-low-birth-weight rates by up to 44 percent.[29] But because WIC provides social services beyond supplemental food, part of these effects may be the result of factors independent of nutrition. Severe malnutrition is clearly not healthy—as data from the Dutch famine study suggest—but it does not appear to be a widespread mechanism connecting economic impoverishment with poor biological outcomes.

Inadequate housing, though another common public health concern, is also not terribly illuminating with regard to low birth weight. In fact, reliable data on housing and low birth weight are rather sparse. For instance, levels of crowding in a given neighborhood have been found to be *negatively* associated with the neighborhood's rates of low birth weight, so that the more crowded the housing in a woman's neighborhood, the less likely she is to give birth to a low-birth-weight infant.[30] This result is quite counterintuitive since one would think that the poor living conditions associated with overcrowding would increase the risk of low birth weight. These data cannot be taken as entirely reliable, however, since neighborhood-level variables like crowding can become terribly confounded with unobserved factors. Evidence connecting housing and infant mortality is stronger than that connecting housing and low birth weight but still not very useful for our purposes. Poor housing has generally been linked to high rates of infant death due to the association between infectious disease and crowding. But the factors contributing to a health phenomenon like infectious disease can be quite distinct from those behind a more general health indicator like birth weight.[31] Thus, while crowding is a major public health concern in general, there is little evidence of its importance in predicting low birth weight.

Access to prenatal care has received a great deal of attention from policy makers, and many government programs since the early 1990s have focused on providing medical services to pregnant women. Yet even here we find mixed evidence. Steven Gortmaker, for instance, found that the relationship between poverty and low birth weight was entirely explained by access to prenatal care.[32] That is, what explained a poor woman's risk for a low-birth-weight birth was not being poor per se but the fact that she was much less likely than her wealthier counterpart to have health insurance. Other studies have found slightly more modest effects of prenatal care—such as a 197-gram increase in average birth weight of babies born to women with adequate prenatal care as compared to women with no prenatal care.[33] Evidence also suggests, however, that prenatal care is not universally effective. Several studies have found that prenatal care is better at increasing black babies' than white babies' birth weights.[34] Other research suggests that income and environment may mediate the effect of prenatal care so that it is least effective in poverty-stricken areas. James Collins and Richard David, for instance, found that prenatal care was effective at lowering black infant mortality only in moderate-income areas.[35]

All of this mixed evidence surrounding questions of impoverishment suggests that a simple, absolute measure of access may not do the trick. Indeed, the relationship between access and health may be quite subtle. As an example, neighborhood characteristics may make it difficult for a poor woman to take full advantage of, say, the health benefits of prenatal care. Evidence suggests that low- and middle-income neighborhoods differ significantly in the services they offer. According to a study cited above, middle-income neighborhoods have proportionally more pharmacies, restaurants, banks, and specialty stores, while low-income neighborhoods had more fast-food restaurants, check-cashing stores, liquor stores, and laundromats. Paying special attention to the availability of adequate nutrition, this study also found that in poor neighborhoods there were four times as many people per food market and that a typical market basket for a family of four costs almost 15 percent more, with produce costing 22 percent more.[36] Such an unequal distribution of services and costs implies that, while poor pregnant women may theoretically be able to gain access to health services (such as pharmacies) or nutrition (at supermarkets), they must make a greater effort to obtain it than their wealthier counterparts. Perhaps neighborhood differences such as these are behind the varying effects of prenatal care cited above. We can imagine that the additional strain and stress that accompany these access barriers may reduce any health benefits associated with prenatal care. As we discussed with regard to race differences in health, context can matter, ultimately determining a resource's meaning or value. A poor woman and a wealthier woman may both be able to visit a pharmacy and a grocery store to obtain the food and vitamins their health care providers recommend. But if the poor woman has to walk ten extra blocks through a dangerous neighborhood or has to wait for the store to order what she needs, the health benefits associated with these resources may well diminish somewhat. The poor woman may even ultimately give up on following her doctor's advice because of all the problems she encounters when trying to do so.

Access to basic necessities is an important part of health. Few would argue that malnutrition, inadequate shelter, or any other form of extreme deprivation is not harmful to a woman and her baby. Yet the denial of basic resources does not seem to account for race and class differences in birth outcomes. Access appears to be a more complicated problem than simply haves versus have-nots. That is, an absolute measure of income does not appear to tell the whole story behind class and health.

BEYOND BASIC NEEDS: RELATIVE INCOME AND PSYCHOSOCIAL FACTORS

If we consider income beyond the dichotomy of poverty versus non-poverty, a more complicated picture of resources emerges. The detailed class differences found in the Whitehall study have been replicated in several different studies in different nations, ranging from the United States to Denmark, Norway, Finland, France, and Japan.[37] Detailed class gradients have even been found in studies of infant mortality.[38] While health differences in some of these countries are less pronounced than those in the United States or Britain, they are still quite notable given that many of these countries have universal health care and lower levels of inequality.

Indeed, the wide variety of contexts across which these linear class effects have been found may make it rather difficult to build simple models of causation. Deprivation of basic necessities, with its close connection to biological outcomes, cannot explain narrow socioeconomic gradients in health. Individuals in middle- and upper-occupational or income categories in the industrialized counties studied above are clearly not being denied the basic necessities that foster health, like food, clothing, and shelter. Even a more nuanced measure of access accounting for quality as well as mere accessibility proves unhelpful in light of historical trends in health care suggesting that health-class relationships are not highly sensitive to changes in quality. As industrialized societies have greatly expanded access to their health care systems over the past 50 years, the use of health care has increased dramatically and has become more equal across social classes. Yet longitudinal data from the United Kingdom show no evidence that such shifts have reduced the mortality gradient.[39] Even as inequalities in quality of care were narrowing, class-based health differences remained stable.

Material explanations of class—such as those found in discussions of access and quality—certainly prove of little help in explaining health differences across a larger number of classes. The diversity of economic situations in these data simply rules out such models. This has led some scholars to abandon the standard material explanation of class for a psychosocial explanation focusing on the relative meaning of class rather than its absolute monetary value. Many authors taking this perspective argue that one's income really has implications for health only because it is higher or lower than someone else's income. While an annual income of $60,000 grants one access to certain biologically necessary resources (like food or housing of varying quality), it also places one in a certain social category that is either above or below another social category. By this logic, one's position vis-à-vis others is what matters. Considering income in such relative terms implies that inequality itself affects health and, as a result, we must pay attention to the whole income distribution, not just those in the lowest income group. Rather than thinking about how many people live below a certain cutoff, here we are concerned with the overall shape of the income distribution. How many people are at the top of the income distribution? How many people are at the bottom? And how much difference is there between the top and the bottom?

There is a fair amount of evidence suggesting that relative class position and overall inequality are important to health. Richard Wilkinson, in an examination of 11 countries, reported a striking relationship between income inequality and life expectancy.[40] According to these results, the proportion of income earned by the least-well-off 70 percent of the population and the overall national inequality index accounted for three-quarters of the variation in life expectancy found across industrialized countries.[41] This approach may prove particularly useful in the United States. One group of researchers comparing inequality across states found that a measure of income distribution called the Robin Hood index (a measure of the proportion of total income that would have to be redistributed from the rich to the poor in order to attain perfect equality of incomes) was strongly related to states' death rates for heart disease, cancers, homicide, and infant mortality.[42] The salience of income inequality in this study is particularly alarming when we note that income inequality in the United States is only getting worse. In 1968 the top 20 percent of U.S. households earned on average $73,754, compared to the $7,202 earned by the bottom 20 percent. In 1994 the average income of the top 20 percent had increased by 44 percent to

$105,945, while the income of the bottom 20 percent had increased by only 7 percent to $7,762.[43] This means that if the degree of income inequality really matters in health outcomes—as these studies suggest—the health of the U.S. population will likely get worse before it gets better.

Focusing on relative class position, while possibly quite fruitful, also currently raises more questions than it answers. For example, what mechanisms and biological pathways may explain this association between relative position and health? When considering access to basic necessities, the mechanism is obvious: if a mother lacks access to food and shelter, she may suffer from malnutrition, exposure, and so on, and such afflictions have an obvious effect on maternal health and birth outcomes. The paths connecting one's position in a status hierarchy to one's health are far less obvious.

Given this lack of clear biological connections in relative models, most authors have focused on psychosocial mechanisms in this debate, arguing that one's social position leads to various psychological conditions (such as stress, self-esteem, feelings of empowerment, etc.) that may in turn affect one's well-being. The evidence most clearly outlining such a relationship, which in fact has sparked most of the current interest in the biological implications of hierarchy, comes from animal populations. Research conducted on nonhuman primates, like baboons and macaques, that live in clearly organized social hierarchies has revealed certain biological pathways connecting social position, stress, and health. Richard Sapolsky has found significant differences between dominant and subordinate males in the functioning of their endocrine systems that appeared to be largely mediated by differences in responses to stress. Testing hormone levels, Sapolsky found that, in dominant males, the physiological response to stress, often referred to as the "fight or flight syndrome," was turned off more rapidly after the stressful event had passed, whereas in subordinate animals the stress response was prolonged.[44] The chronic stress experienced by these subordinate baboons can have definitive health implications because hormones released during times of stress divert the body's resources away from health-promoting functions like growth, tissue repair, and the immune system.[45] Thus, according to these findings, low-ranking animals are sicker because animals on the bottom experience more stress and the more stress an animal experiences, the less time its body spends healing and maintaining itself.

We cannot directly apply Sapolsky's findings to our research since such work has not been replicated with human subjects. The intrusiveness of the physiological testing is by most standards ethically unaccept-able for human subjects. However, comparable evidence suggests that social position and stress are linked to poor human health as well. For instance, Michael Marmot has found that, on average, people at all occu-pational ranks in Britain have elevated blood pressure when at work. But blood pressure drops much more when at home for those in higher-ranked positions than for those in lower-ranked positions.[46] Much like the primates in Sapolsky's studies, those at the top of the hierarchy recover from stress more quickly than those at the bottom. These stress-based explanations of health differences do seem to suggest that social positions have inherent health-promoting or health-hindering qualities, and it may be that, the greater the difference between the top and the bottom, the greater the health differences between groups.

With regard to low birth weight, stress-based explanations have also received some support. A number of studies have found that pregnant women experiencing stressors have an elevated risk of delivering a low-birth-weight infant.[47] To date, most evidence suggests that this connec-tion works through preterm delivery, such that stress leads to low birth weight by inducing early labor.[48] Stress is assumed to raise corticos-teroids (a hormone related to stress) in pregnant women,[49] which are supposed to make the "clock" for delivery run faster.[50] Authors have also found that attributes protecting against stress, such as high levels of social support, are less effective for women in low-income areas,[51] so that these connections between stress and low birth weight may be the most pronounced among poor women.

While the stress paradigm has received a great deal of attention and a fair amount of empirical support, it has also been criticized for detract-ing attention from the primary factor of these models—social position. Bruce Link has argued that "research on the biological consequences of stress . . . is seen as an exciting new development . . . interest has fol-lowed the most recent step in the progression toward disease outcomes, while concern with the earlier foci has dissipated."[52] In other words, as new developments have emerged, researchers have paid more attention to the biological specifics of stress than to the question of why social position is so strongly related to stress in the first place. Offering an alternative to the stress paradigm, Link has proposed the fundamental cause hypothesis outlined previously in this chapter. Similar to the stress hypothesis, the fundamental cause hypothesis suggests that rela-tive social positions have inherent qualities that may promote or hinder health. Rather than pointing to inherent levels of stress, however, Link suggests that social positions provide people with resources like knowledge, money, power, and prestige that can be used to obtain health resources. "As new risk factors become apparent," Link writes, "people of higher socioeconomic status are more favorably situated to know about the risks and have the resources that allow them to engage in protective efforts to avoid them."[53] For example, some authors have suggested that during the 1960s, when evidence of the risks of smoking began to emerge, a new class pattern developed in these behaviors. There is no evidence that, prior to the 1960s, rates of smoking were higher among lower socioeconomic groups. However, during the 1960s individuals of higher socioeconomic status were more likely to quit smoking, and research on current populations finds strong socioeconomic gradients in smoking behavior.[54] In other words, wealthier people learned about the heath risks of smoking more quickly than poorer people and could then mobilize resources to more effectively change their behavior.

Ambiguity in the research on low birth weight that we have outlined so far may indeed be clarified by considering fundamental power differences within hierarchies. For instance, variations in the impact of poverty by race and in the effectiveness of prenatal care by both race and class may occur because one's relative social position allows one to acquire and take advantage of knowledge to different degrees. A black woman in poverty may face racial discrimination in addition to financial barriers, and thus she may be in a particularly disadvantaged position as compared to a poor white woman in her efforts to alter behavior. Similarly, while both poor and middle-class women may use prenatal care, the poor woman may face significant barriers not confronted by the middle-class woman (such as the neighborhood differences discussed above) in following through on the doctor's advice. Thus, when we consider income as a relative measure, the resources and knowledge tied to one's social position become primary causes of class-based health differences, and individual conditions and behaviors (like stress or prenatal care) are meaningful only in the context of larger social hierarchies.

It is important to note, though, that the relative income approach to health has not gone unchallenged. There is great variety in how authors have measured inequality, and some critics have suggested that individual investigators chose indicators based on whether or not they supported the relative income hypothesis. Other authors have argued that failure to adjust inequality measures for taxes, household size, and transfer payments may have exaggerated the effect of inequality on health.[55] An alternative criticism is that the relationship between inequality and health may be a statistical artifact.[56] As we discussed earlier in this chapter, evidence of income's nonlinear effect on health suggests that income has a stronger positive effect on health if one is below the national poverty line than if one is above it. Another way to put this is that being deprived has a very strong negative effect on health, while being privileged has a relatively weak positive effect on health. When researchers start comparing very large groups, like countries, this non-linear effect of income on health begins to cause problems (technically referred to as ecological fallacies or aggregation bias). There will likely be more people below the poverty line in an economically heterogeneous country than in an economically more homogeneous country, which means that the strong negative effects of deprivation will pull the heterogeneous nation's average health downward (since the comparatively weak effect of privilege will fail to counteract them). This criticism of inequality arguments implies that there are no inherent qualities in social position that affect health. Rather, according to this argument, the nation's health simply depends on the absolute number of people who are deprived of basic necessities. The evidence on these various positions, in sum, is mixed.[57]

ALTERNATIVE FRAMEWORKS: BIOLOGY AS A CAUSAL FACTOR

Throughout all the studies we have reviewed so far in this chapter, there is a common assumption—that social conditions are *causing* class differences in health. While the research discussed above may vary in terms of how authors measured income or which specific mediating pathways they focused on, it all assumes that the socioeconomic phenomenon of income, class, or status is a causal factor and that the biological phenomenon of health status is a result. This is certainly a plausible explanation for the association between health and class but is far from the only possibility.

As we discussed earlier, reverse causation is a common hazard in health research. That is, rather than class causing health status, health may be determining socioeconomic status. This reverse scenario has not received as much empirical attention as models of economic causation. In some respects, arguments of biological causation seem to have fallen through the disciplinary cracks—social scientists with sympathies for and data on social position are often not interested in biology as a cause, while biologists with sympathies for and data on physical conditions are often not interested in social position. At the same time, this potential for reverse causation has remained a problem lurking behind many studies of inequality and health. Indeed, it is quite easy to imagine how reverse scenarios might work. If afflicted with an illness, one has more difficulty attending school and work, making it harder to acquire human capital. This mechanism may refer not simply to the number of sick days but to one's underlying health potentials or compositions that, say, give one more energy or motivation and facilitate acquiring economic capital.

In the association between class and infant health several biological conditions may be at work. For instance, pregnancy-related complications, such as anemia and abnormal blood pressure, may hinder fetal development and lead to elevated risks of low birth weight.[58] Shorter maternal stature and younger age are also biological characteristics that increase chances of low birth weight.[59] And, as is documented in the previous chapter, parents having been born low birth weight themselves are an important biological factor that predicts the risk of low birth weight. However, as we might expect, such biological risk factors are not randomly distributed across the population but, rather, vary systematically by class. Poor pregnant women compared to their wealthier counterparts are more likely to suffer pregnancy-related complications that might lead to low birth weight, are more likely to be young, and are more likely to be of short stature. Similarly, poor parents are significantly more likely than better-off parents to have been born low birth weight.

The association among teenage pregnancy, low birth weight, and low socioeconomic status can offer us a more detailed picture of these social-biological mix-ups. Some authors have argued that young maternal age lowers birth weight through biological mechanisms because the fetus is in competition for nutrients still needed by the growing adolescent mother.[60] Other authors have argued that young maternal age may result in slow biological adaptation to pregnancy (e.g., weight gain, placental development), which places the fetus at greater risk for growth retardation.[61] While such biological processes may certainly place a fetus at risk, it is not so clear that they really cause low birth weight among young mothers. Teenage mothers are overwhelmingly concentrated below the poverty line, both before and after their pregnancies, and poverty often plays a crucial role in a young woman's chances of becoming pregnant and bringing a baby to term.[62] Alternatively, therefore, socioeconomic status may be the true causal factor, and age may simply be a proxy.

For example, Arline Geronimus has argued that teenage childbearing is brought about by poverty because it is a rational response to the conditions of low socioeconomic status. Life expectancies in poor communities are quite short—researchers have found that more than one-third of women living in Harlem or in Chicago's Southside die by age 65 and little more than half of men in these neighborhoods can expect to survive to age 55.[63] (Such figures are quite striking in comparison to the national life expectancy of 79.5 for women and 73.8 for men.[64]) According to Geronimus, such poor survival prospects makes early childbearing appear quite rational for people living in poverty. Geronimus writes, "If one believes that responsible parenting includes maximizing the chances that a parent will survive to see and help her children grow up, then insecurity about one's longevity would be a serious consideration when contemplating whether to defer childbearing."[65] Poverty may, thus, alter living conditions so extensively that early childbearing becomes a comparatively attractive prospect for poor young people. And here we see our causal dilemma. If we as researchers encountered a group of pregnant teenagers and examined them thoroughly, we would likely find that they faced both biological and economic risk factors for low birth weight. But since we had just met these teenagers and the multiple risk factors they faced were already in place, we would not be able to tell what was responsible for their high-risk profiles. Their biological risk profiles could be the causal agent, but so could their social risk profiles. Because social and biological risk tend to go together, data covering only short periods of time can make sorting out causation difficult.

However, considering a scenario that covers a longer period of time— say, generations—we may indeed be able to sort out social and biological causation. Examining Figure 3.1, we see that certain patterns of effects across two generations will reveal either biological or economic causation in patterns of birth weight and socioeconomic status. Considering first the set of inner arrows in the figure, we find that neither maternal nor filial birth weight has any effect on socioeconomic status. Rather, in this scenario maternal adult socioeconomic status (along with maternal birth weight) determines filial birth weight. Meanwhile, the adult socioeconomic status of the child is determined by the mother's adult socioeconomic status—we find no biological determinants of class but rather an economic inheritance of class. Using data that span a long period of time and that imply a certain ordering

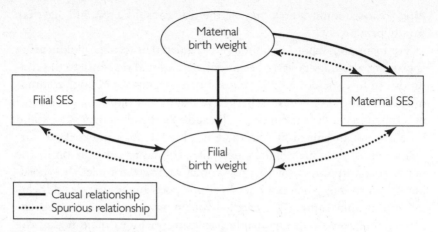

Figure 3.1. Intergenerational patterns of causation. Outer arrows trace the pattern of infant health causing adult socioeconomic status (SES). Inner arrows trace the pattern of SES causing infant health.

of outcomes can, of course, alternatively reveal biological causation. Looking at the outer set of arrows in Figure 3.1, we see that birth weight plays a key causal role. Not only does maternal birth weight determine maternal adult socioeconomic status, but this pattern is replicated across generations as well, so that filial birth weight determines filial adult socioeconomic status (net of the effects of maternal adult socioeconomic status). At the same time, maternal socioeconomic status has no direct causal link in this model to the biological outcome of filial birth weight but only an effect on filial adult socioeconomic status (independent of the effects of filial birth weight).

In these hypothetical cases of low birth weight, we are able to isolate causal roles for economics and infant health precisely because there is an assumed temporal ordering to these variables. In the case of teen pregnancy cited above, we noted biological and social risk, but because we had no information on which of these risks had been established first, we had no clear way to determine which was elevating the risk of low birth weight. Here, in contrast, we know that maternal birth weight had to have preceded maternal adult socioeconomic status and that filial birth weight had to have preceded filial adult socioeconomic status. Consequently, a relationship among these variables (found in the outer set of arrows) would imply biological causation. Similarly, we know that maternal adult socioeconomic status preceded filial birth weight, and so a relationship between these variables (found in the inner set of arrows) implies economic causation.

Beyond pure biological or social causation, however, there also exists the further possibility of biosocial interactions determining socioeconomic status and birth weight. It may be the case that social and biological factors are not operating separately but rather are more intricately related so that they interact with one another or depend on one another. In the case of such an interaction effect, parental birth weight and parental socioeconomic status may have a multiplicative effect that creates particularly high or low risks of low birth weight. An initial risk factor, like parental low birth weight status—to the extent that it is biologically determined—may be buffered by additional income that allows for a better diet or for special prenatal care. Alternatively, of course, the environment may exacerbate biological risks. Barbara Starfield and her colleagues, for example, have shown that a family tendency toward low birth weight (in the form of an older sibling having been born low birth weight—which may or may not have genetic causes) interacts with poverty status to create a subset of poor women who are at particularly high risk for giving birth to a low-birth-weight baby.[66] Biology and society can become intertwined not only in their relative effects on one another but also in a cumulative fashion creating particular subsets of risk. Most of the research we have addressed in this chapter has focused on either biology or society, limiting analysis to the separate causal paths outlined in Figures 3.1. However, in the analyses that follow in this and the next chapter, we will attempt to consider multiple causal factors that may operate and interact with one another over time.

RESEARCH QUESTIONS AND STATISTICAL APPROACH

In the following analysis we investigate the first half of our intergenerational model, addressing the question, Do the income and other socioeconomic conditions of a mother during her pregnancy affect her chances of having a low birth weight infant after taking into account her own birth weight, the father's birth weight, and other, unobserved family-related factors? We also test for a situation in which a family tendency may interact with environment by posing the question, does the effect of the mother's socioeconomic conditions during pregnancy depend on her family's birth weight history?

As in the previous chapter, we use a combination of between-family and within-family comparison techniques to address these questions. First, comparing low birth weight across a random sample of families, we examine the effects of maternal socioeconomic characteristics on filial low birth weight, holding parental low birth weight and the above variables constant. In these models, any residual effect of socioeconomic status after controls are in place can be assumed to operate independently of an intergenerational family propensity for low birth weight. However, in these analyses we will again be unable to rule out unobserved variable bias or spuriousness. There are a host of unobserved characteristics that affect both filial birth weight and maternal socioeconomic status, including but not limited to overall parental health status, genetic endowments, class or social status, and environmental conditions. Therefore, in the models that follow we cannot be certain that, say, our income effects have not been inflated due to the poor general health status of low-income parents.

In order to address this potential spuriousness, we again use family fixed-effects models to factor out unobserved variation—but this time we compare siblings rather than cousins. This is a very strict statistical test that factors out, for the most part, unobserved variation in parental characteristics and home environment across families. We choose to use this technique of sibling comparisons in this chapter because we have the luxury of access to income data prior to each pregnancy by the same mother. By contrast, when we were interested in the effect of parental low birth weight in chapter 2, we had to compare across two parents (who were sisters) and track the effect of a change in parental biological contributions. Therefore, as shown in Figure 3.2, variation in socioeconomic status in these analyses is a question of variation between two pregnancies or points in time. A mother being in poverty, married, or over age 18 during one pregnancy but not another will be captured in this analysis, but variation between different mothers will be held constant.

In this approach of sibling comparisons, behavioral factors will be a potential bias only to the extent that they vary between two pregnancies and are related to changes in income that occur between pregnancies. For instance, if between her first and second pregnancy a mother suffered a loss of income and began to behave differently, we may face behavioral bias—in this case, new habits rather than the drop in income may account for the low birth weight of the second baby. But if behavioral changes are a response to a change in income, they may—to the

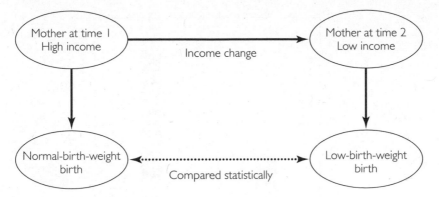

Figure 3.2. Sibling fixed-effects model, part I

degree they determine birth weight—be mediating an income effect rather than playing a causal role. However, if a behavioral change precedes the change in income, it is possible that behavior is playing a causal role in both the income fluctuation and the birth outcome. Thus in the case of sibling comparisons, the behavioral change is a potential bias only if it falls in between two pregnancies and is preceded by a change in income.

THE IMPORTANCE OF SOCIOECONOMIC CONDITIONS

We cannot find an effect of income in our analysis when we consider income a completely independent risk factor. In short, it appears statistically meaningless when we factor out the overall effects of the mother and a small number of time-sensitive confounding factors.[67] This holds true whether we compare across families or across siblings within the same family. That said, the negligible effects of income that we have documented so far still leave open the possibility that they depend on biology. That is, the effect of income on birth weight may differ according to whether or not a parent was born low birth weight. We address this hypothesis in Figure 3.3 by including appropriate interaction terms in our regression model and by separating the fixed-effects analyses into two models—one referring only to children who had a low-birth-weight parent and the other to those who did not.

According to this figure, income's effects on low birth weight do indeed depend on a biological legacy. Factoring out the effects of various control variables but allowing parental birth weight to interact (see

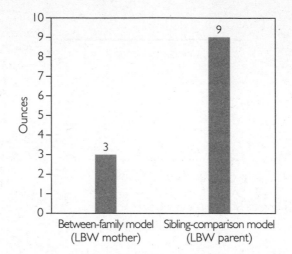

Figure 3.3. The impact of income and parental low birth weight on filial low birth weight (LBW): the number of ounces added to birth weight by a unit increase in the income-to-needs ratio among babies with an LBW parent, using between-family and sibling-comparison models. See appendix B, Table 3.1, for descriptive statistics related to these variables; Table 3.2 for subsample characteristics; Table 3.3 (columns 3 and 4, respectively) for regression coefficients related to this analysis. (OLS, ordinary least squares)

the left-hand bar), income has a modest effect for those born to women who were of low birth weight themselves, increasing birth weight by approximately three ounces for each unit increase in the ratio of income to the poverty line (or the income-to-needs ratio). In our sibling comparisons (represented by the right-hand bar), we split the sample according to whether the infant had a low-birth-weight parent and find that, if a child is at medical risk (i.e., has a low-birth-weight parent), then he or she benefits substantially from increases in income. For each unit increase in a family's income-to-needs ratio, a child's birth weight rises by more than half a pound (nine ounces)—as compared to his or her siblings.[68] Thus, additional income appears to have beneficial effects for those babies at the greatest biological risk.

While this result likely does point to specific benefits we can expect from income, it also must be noted that biological or etiological differences in the previous generation may present an alternative story. Low birth weight, depending on whether it is the result of a premature birth or growth retardation, can have varying health implications.[69] In some cases, low birth weight leads to serious impairments that hinder a person's economic potential, while in other cases, its effects are not so serious. To the extent that the heritability of birth weight varies by etiological differences that imply different long-term implications for socioeconomic status, this interaction between biological legacy and income may really be the result of parallel patterns across the implications and heritability of low birth weight. That is, if mothers with less serious forms of low birth weight are less likely to pass low-birth-weight status on to their children and are also less likely to falter economically, we may find this pattern in which additional income (serving in this case as a proxy for a less serious form of parental low birth weight) reduces the likelihood of a low-birth-weight birth in light of a biological legacy. But in this scenario, such a pattern would imply not the biosocial interaction that we have assumed but rather a complicated pattern of biological causation affecting heritability and parental development patterns. Since we have no information on the etiology of birth weight in our data (or on the specific heritability of each etiology), we cannot speak directly to this alternative, and it does indeed remain a potential confounding issue. That said, however, there is a great deal of evidence documenting the protective effects of income during pregnancy, which further supports our interpretation of a biosocial interaction.[70]

CONCLUSION

A family history of low birth weight is clearly a very important predictor of low birth weight, and our findings challenge earlier studies documenting the crucial role of socioeconomic status in birth outcomes. However, our results do not suggest that biological histories can wholly account for variation in low birth weight. Rather, our interaction terms point to the importance of simultaneously examining social and biological factors when considering the distribution of health across populations. Minorities and low-income individuals are at high risk for low-birth-weight births as compared to nonminority and higher-income individuals. One's risk of low birth weight is, furthermore, very sensitive to a biological predisposition (that is, having a family history of low birth weight). However, these two facts do not necessarily imply that minorities and low-income individuals are more likely to be biologically predisposed toward low birth weight. Biological predispositions toward low birth weight or another health condition may be equally distributed throughout the population. However, since the economic resources that may buffer a predisposition are not equally distributed, we find unequal patterns in the risk. As one author writes, "the important point is that genes determine who may get sick within a class, but environmental factors determine the frequency of sickness."[71] If we were again to take 100 high-income couples and 100 low-income couples, we might find that 20 of the couples in each income group were biologically predisposed toward low birth weight. However, if each of these couples then had a baby, we might find that only 4 of the predisposed high-income couples had a low-birth-weight baby, while 17 of the predisposed low-income couples had a low-birth-weight baby. The high-income couples likely had the resources (e.g., better nutrition, better prenatal care) to counteract biological tendencies, while the lower-income couples likely did not. Therefore, to suggest that there is a large, biologically heritable component of birth weight is not to imply that biology is destiny and is wholly responsible for patterns of birth weight across populations. Rather, it is more likely the case that society and biology work in tandem to produce inequalities in health across generations.

CHAPTER 4

Is Biology Destiny?

*Birth Weight, Infant Mortality,
and Educational Achievement*

A simple child,
That lightly draws its breath,
And feels its life in every limb,
What should it know of death?
   William Wordsworth,
   We Are Seven (1798)

Improvements in medical technology are forcing many physicians, policy makers, and parents to reconsider the meaning of a low-birth-weight
birth. As neonatal intensive care units (NICUs) have become better
equipped to help low-weight babies and as a greater number of high-
risk deliveries are carried out in tertiary centers, the survival rates for
low-birth-weight infants have improved dramatically. Over the past
20 years, all birth weight–specific survival rates have improved notably;
however, the most significant improvement has been in the survival rates
of the smallest babies. In 1961 a baby born weighing between 1,001
and 1,500 grams (a very-low-birth-weight baby) had about a 50 percent
chance of surviving its first year of life, while today such a baby has
more than a 90 percent chance of survival. Babies born weighing even
less, between 751 grams and 1,000 grams, today enjoy a greater than
75 percent chance of survival.[1]

While such reductions in birth weight–specific mortality are a significant accomplishment, they also raise complicated ethical questions.
For one thing, they force us to consider the "quality" of survival and
the long-term implications of low birth weight. Very-low-birth-weight
infants often can be kept alive only under extreme forms of medical
intervention. In some cases, special liquids have to be pumped into

newborn lungs so that they can breathe. In other cases, steroids are used to force the lungs to mature faster.[2] Unfortunately for many of these fragile babies, the long-term prognosis is quite poor. Early health complications and interventions can have cognitive and physical effects that may last a lifetime. More and more frequently, doctors, parents, and hospitals are faced with difficult choices about whether to keep the most vulnerable infants alive, and often there are disturbing conflicts. For instance, there are cases where parents' wish to let their ailing child die peacefully has run up against hospital policies of resuscitating all babies above a certain weight. One such case involved Sydney, an infant born at just 22 weeks. After watching her suffer for a few days on life support, the parents decided to let her pass away in her mother's arms. Hospital procedure, however, forced physicians to resuscitate the child. At the age of ten, Sydney remained unable to walk and had undergone 13 operations to remove fluid from her brain. When interviewed by the media about his daughter, the father voiced his frustration with the hospital, complaining that his "daughter suffers the consequences of their medical experimentation each day."[3]

That is the paradox of the issue. Because low-birth-weight infants are now more likely to survive thanks to medical technology, they are also more likely to be confronted with multiple health and developmental deficiencies.[4] At the earliest stages, often while still in the NICU, low-weight infants face a high risk of several complications including severe asphyxia, neonatal meningitis, symptomatic intercranial hemorrhage, and neonatal seizures. Once out of the NICU, a broad spectrum of cognitive and behavioral problems remains. Scores on both verbal IQ (a test of cognitive and language skills) and performance IQ (a test of motor-perceptual skills) generally are lower with lower birth weights.[5] Low-birth-weight children can also exhibit more erratic behavior than non-low-birth-weight children and may have greater trouble with social interaction and emotional expression.[6] Even when such conditions are not severe, they still warrant concern—mild levels of such problems can interfere with normal academic and social progress. For instance, studies have found that low-birth-weight (LBW) children have more trouble behaving in school than non-LBW children and are more likely than their normal-birth-weight counterparts to repeat an early grade.[7]

It is often assumed that the effects of low birth weight dwindle with age. Physicians generally take gestational age into account in making diagnoses for only the first few years of a child's life, and most researchers track the effects of birth weight and prematurity only until around age 12. However, recent evidence suggests that birth weight may have lifelong effects. A group of researchers in Denmark found that the average cognitive functioning (IQ) of 18-year-old male draftees was significantly lower if the individual had been born low birth weight.[8] Following a group of children born in 1970 until they reached age 26, some British researchers found that adults who had been born low birth weight were only half as likely as adults born of normal weight to have professional or managerial jobs.[9] Recent data from the United States collected by Maureen Hack and her colleagues similarly reveal that, at age 20, very-low-birth-weight individuals are less likely to have graduated high school and are more likely to be chronically ill than normal-birth-weight individuals.[10] Finally, another study following a cohort of female nurses found that low birth weight was associated with higher rates of cardiovascular disease in adulthood.[11]

Because the lasting effects of low birth weight have begun to receive attention only since the late 1980s, there is still a fair amount of debate over the best way to study these effects. It can be quite complicated to isolate and effectively measure the effects of low birth weight as distinguished from the other health and social risk factors with which it is associated. For instance, the study by Hack and her colleagues cited above finds low-birth-weight effects that are somewhat smaller than those found elsewhere. This lower magnitude could mean that low birth weight is not as significant as some evidence has suggested or could be a result of how these researchers designed their study. To begin with, these researchers use what could be considered a "loose" definition of high school graduation, counting anyone who ever gets a degree—even an equivalency degree—as a high school graduate. Since it has been well documented that equivalency degrees are not as valuable in the job market as high school diplomas,[12] this decision to count all degrees as equal could significantly reduce differences in educational attainment and its long-term implications. A recent response by Hack and her colleagues to this critique, though, has bolstered their initial results by showing that differences in graduation rates by birth weight remain small (and, in fact, are statistically insignificant) even when all those with equivalency degrees are excluded from the study.[13]

However, the small effects of low birth weight found in this study could alternatively result from the sample used, which consisted exclusively of poor babies born in Cleveland. Since all the children in this study—low birth weight and normal birth weight alike—are living in or close to poverty, high school graduation rates will already be significantly below national averages. This means that, when considering the effects of birth weight, these researchers are already working at the lower end of the distribution, where graduation rates may not have much farther to fall. In other words, low birth weight may have only a minimal effect in this study because environmental conditions have so significantly limited children's future prospects that the effect of biology is hindered. In other economic conditions, low birth weight may matter quite a bit more.

Our data include whether a child was born low birth weight and whether he or she was born into poverty, so we can factor out each of these "effects"—but only to the degree that these "effects" are unbiased by differences we may not know about. Using our technique of sibling comparisons, however, we can take care of further potential biases without anticipating each one specifically. That is, we can factor out many unobserved differences between low-birth-weight and normal-birth-weight children and between wealthier and poorer families that may be causing spurious social or biological patterns in traditional models. In this chapter, we use these methods to uncover social and biological stories of causation by considering how one's low birth weight and poverty statuses in early childhood determine chances of graduating from high school in a timely fashion (i.e., by the end of the 19th year of life). To make sure, however, that the effects of low birth weight we uncover are not limited to the single measure of timely graduation, we also assess whether birth weight matters to additional measures of educational progress—namely, having to repeat a grade, being enrolled in special education, or being classified as learning disabled. We then use comparisons of the birth weights of twin sets to factor out even more unobserved differences. Even when comparing the effects of birth weight differences between singleton siblings, we cannot know whether it is the effect of prematurity, birth weight, or some other health or congenital problem for which weight is acting as a proxy that really matters. Further, we cannot know the extent to which birth weight is acting as a proxy for unobserved social conditions that may vary between pregnancies and that may affect both birth weight and its apparent "consequences," thereby causing spurious effects. Twin differences in birth weight hold constant gestational age and the social and health conditions surrounding the pregnancy. Identical twin comparisons further factor out genetic differences between the siblings. There are, of course, complicating issues surrounding the use of twins, and we will address these later in the chapter.

If we combine this analysis with that in chapter 3, we can begin to piece together an intergenerational cycle of social and/or biological inheritance. We saw in the last chapter that a baby's well-being at birth is determined by the biological and social conditions of her parents. We will now show that a baby's well-being at birth goes on to affect her chances of survival and prosperity down the road. If a low-birth-weight baby then grows up to have her own child, the biological and social conditions of multiple generations are interacting to shape this baby's welfare. By tracing such family patterns over long periods of time and by using stringent methods of comparison, we can begin to sort out the *direction* of social and biological inequality. If we look at socioeconomic gradients in health at only one point in time, it is unclear whether people are sick because they are poor, or they are poor because they are sick. However, when we begin to consider the transmission of characteristics from one generation to the next, the pathways of cause and effect become clearer, and the mechanisms that maintain social and biological inequalities over time are revealed.

LOW BIRTH WEIGHT AND CHANCES FOR ADULT SUCCESS: BIOLOGICAL CAUSATION

Low birth weights (particularly those below 1,500 grams) are associated with a host of serious biological conditions that could clearly account for poor adult outcomes. Major neurological handicaps occur two to four times more frequently in low-birth-weight and premature babies than in normal-birth-weight full-term infants and may include cerebral palsy, mental retardation, hearing loss, and visual impairment.[14] Lower respiratory infections, like bronchiolitis and pneumonia, are also quite common among LBW infants[15] and can frequently lead to chronic lung disease, which limits children's activities for years.[16] Gastrointestinal problems are also common among LBW premature infants and can often mean that infants have trouble absorbing nutrients from food, making it even harder for already vulnerable babies to thrive and grow.[17] In some cases, these gastrointestinal problems may also lead to chronic conditions—like "short gut" syndrome (problems related to having half or more of the small intestine removed) and intestinal strictures (narrowing of the intestine that may lead to blockage).[18] Finally, LBW infants are also frequently afflicted with cardiovascular sequelae, including persistent patent ductus arteriosus (an opening in the pulmonary artery) and chronic hypertension.[19] In many cases, disabilities such as these mean that children cannot progress at the same rate as their peers and must be placed in special education programs, or that they are frequently absent from school and are held back a grade. In either case, the connections between low birth weight, disability, and difficulty in school are quite apparent.

When low birth weight is less severe (usually when a birth weight falls between 1,500 and 2,500 grams), the connections between birth weight and school progress become less obvious and arguments of biological causation may not be so immediately convincing. The majority of LBW infants do not suffer readily apparent handicaps—such as cerebral palsy, mental retardation, or blindness—but rather exhibit more subtle abnormalities that cause them to lag behind their normal-birth-weight counterparts at most stages of development.[20] In many cases, boys in this weight range suffer more than similarly sized girls. As we discussed in chapter 1, the entire birth weight distribution of girls is shifted toward lighter weights, so it is possible that the range of unhealthy weights for girls is lower than that for boys. It has also been argued, however, that these differences in the implications of low birth weight (particularly differences in the rates and severity of behavioral problems) have to do with differences in the ways that parents treat LBW boys compared to LBW girls.

Beginning in infancy, LBW babies (boys and girls alike) generally require more familiarization time before they can recognize people or things, implying that they are not processing visual information as quickly or in the same way as larger babies.[21] Low-birth-weight infants also frequently have more trouble than normal-birth-weight infants manipulating objects.[22] Such subtle differences—ones that many parents may not even notice—can still set the stage for future problems. Since exploring by touch and watching visual queues are the main ways that babies learn, these seemingly small deficiencies can act cumulatively, causing LBW babies to fall behind in later intellectual development.[23] One study, for instance, found that at 30 months of age there was a nine-point difference in IQ between low-birth-weight and normal-birth-weight babies; however, at 48 months this gap had grown to fifteen points.[24] (Although there is not a full-scale IQ test for children this young, researchers often approximate it using portions of the exam.) Subtle cognitive abnormalities, resulting from low birth weight and having a cumulative effect on IQ, are certainly a possible biological explanation for LBW children's tendency to face academic risk. One study found that by ages 8 to 10 low-birth-weight children are twice as likely as normal-birth-weight children to fall into the borderline IQ category that is usually associated with special education needs.[25]

Low-birth-weight children also display higher rates of behavioral problems, which may blur the line between biological and environmental factors.[26] At infancy, premature infants cry more, are less soothable, and tend to change behavioral states more frequently than their full-term counterparts. This shifting behavior, while it may seem simple fussing, can be quite detrimental since it may make it harder for LBW infants and their caregivers to interact in positive ways. Several studies have found that mother-infant interactions are less positive and stimulating when the baby is low birth weight. When interacting with their mothers, low-birth-weight infants are generally less responsive—they vocalize less, make eye contact less frequently, and do not play with their mothers as often as normal-birth-weight babies. Correspondingly, studies have found that mothers of low-birth-weight infants exhibit fewer happy expressions when interacting with their babies than do mothers of normal-birth-weight infants.[27] A great deal of evidence has suggested that positive and frequent infant-caregiver interactions are crucial to normal development,[28] and therefore inadequate interactions with the caregiver at early ages (because of behavioral problems resulting from low birth weight) could be an alternative mechanism—crossing biological and social lines—that accounts for IQ differences between low-birth-weight and normal-birth-weight children. When mothers are poor—as many mothers of LBW infants are—these behavioral aspects of low birth weight could be even more problematic. Experiencing greater stress or perhaps having their own cognitive or behavioral problems, poor mothers tend to have fewer positive interactions with their children—regardless of the child's birth weight status.[29] Thus, when a poor mother has an LBW child who is less responsive than other children, positive interactions may be particularly lacking, making it rather unlikely that this child will develop at a normal rate.

This collection of evidence points us toward no single explanation for the potential effects of low birth weight on educational attainment. Since there are so many conditions associated with low birth weight—each of which can place a child at risk individually, and all of which can act cumulatively to create an entire risk profile—finding a consistent story to account for the connection between low birth weight and low educational attainment can be rather difficult. This difficulty may indeed suggest the need for a more general approach to low birth weight. Rather than treating low birth weight as a specific health condition with a particular set of mechanisms for determining life chances, we may be better off considering it as a proxy for overall health constitution. As noted previously, low birth weight can be caused by a host of underlying conditions—ranging from nutritional deficits, to blood volume, to the fetus's position in the womb. And since the majority of cases of low birth weight cannot be tied to a particular cause (and are thus idiopathic in nature), low birth weight is in fact frequently treated as a general indicator of infant or maternal health, rather than a specific health condition. (Again, we will address this issue with the analysis of twin differences later in the chapter.)

Further, there is a tradition in health and inequality research that treats size (specifically, height) as a proxy for general health status, and evidence surrounding low birth weight can fit nicely within this framework. Tall people are more likely than short people to move up the social ladder. It was for a long time assumed that tall people found it easier to excel because their shorter peers looked up to and respected them. When it was discovered, however, that childhood height is a stronger predictor of adult socioeconomic mobility than adult height,[30] this explanation of tall people getting treated differently was largely rejected, since one's employer, coworkers, and the like probably do not respect one for having been tall as a seven-year-old. (Although short children are more likely to become short adults and tall children, tall adults, people grow at different enough speeds that not all short adults were necessarily short children, and not all tall adults were necessarily tall children. Childhood and adult heights are therefore independent enough phenomena that this study does not merely reflect adult height-class associations.) Given such childhood evidence, most people now assume that associations between adult height and class are reflections of something in childhood (namely, health) that affects both height and future social mobility. There is a fair amount of evidence supporting this claim, suggesting that taller people are healthier than shorter people and that these taller-healthier people are more likely than their shorter-sicker counterparts to climb the social ladder.[31]

Recent evidence has suggested that birth weight—an alternative measure of size—may play an important role in this connection between height and economic attainment. Jere Behrman and Mark Rosenzweig—using female twins to hold genetic variation and uterine conditions constant—trace the effects of birth status on height and class. According to this study, weight at birth is a strong predictor of both height and class. Comparing only genetically identical twins, these authors find that every additional pound at birth increases adult height by more than half an inch (0.6 inches to be exact). Birth weight, furthermore, has a strong effect on educational attainment and adult income, so that every additional pound at birth enjoyed by a twin results in almost a third of a year more of school and a 7 percent increase in adult earnings.[32] Thus, birth weight in this study seems to be important to both height and to later attainment. To the degree that we accept the hypothesis that height reflects underlying health constitutions, these results could be interpreted to mean that birth weight determines health and later attainment or that birth weight determines later attainment through the mechanism of underlying health status.

Birth weight and height in this particular study cannot be the result of genetic differences, since these authors are comparing the birth weights of genetically identical twins. However, as our results have suggested so far, there are significant reasons to suspect that there is a genetic component to birth weight in the larger, nontwin population. And researchers have found that up to 80 percent of the variation in height may be due to genetics.[33] Therefore, to the degree that birth weight and height in nontwins are the result of genetics, we may see a pattern in which genetics determines health and health determines life chances. If parents pass size on to their children through their genes and if size then plays an important role in economic attainment, genetics could play a very large role in our chances for future success.

This approach that considers birth weight to be indicative of an underlying condition—be it genetic or nongenetic—refocuses our attention away from specific mechanisms or pathways to the measure of size itself. This switch does not, however, avoid the problem of contradictory evidence and alternative social explanation. There are several reasons to be suspicious of arguments that connect size to inherent health conditions. A significant body of evidence suggests that social and economic conditions in infancy and childhood play a strong role in determining childhood and adult height. Data from the antebellum period in the United States and from contemporary industrializing nations suggest that adults' height is quite sensitive to the levels of nutritional access and urbanization that they experience during infancy.[34] Such connections between height and socioeconomic conditions have been found in the contemporary United States as well. Sanders Korenman and Jane Miller find that poor kids in the United States are almost 8 percent more likely than wealthy kids to be short for their ages.[35] In this study, Korenman and Miller factor out the effects of birth weight

(which, the Behrman and Rosenzweig study suggests, is related to adult
height) and use cousin comparisons to reduce the influence of genetic
differences. It is therefore relatively unlikely that childhood height in
this study reflects innate characteristics. Rather, these results imply that
parents' incomes also matter in the health-height equation.

Other evidence suggests a psychosocial explanation of childhood
height and class. For example, a Swedish study that asked adults about
their childhood conditions found that shorter people had suffered not
only economic hardship as children but often domestic conflict as well.[36]
Another study—more convincing because it factors out the effects of
parents' height and tracks growth across childhood—similarly finds
that family conflict is associated with particularly slow growth.[37] As we
discuss in chapter 3, stress can divert the body's resources away from
functions that are not immediately necessary—such as growth—and
so environmental conditions, not inherent characteristics, could also
account for stature. It is, further, not hard to imagine that these negative conditions associated with short stature (that is, poverty and
domestic conflict) could also lead people to have more trouble at school
and work. Thus, here we see environmental conditions that could also
account for the connection between height and mobility. While there is
no evidence on this point, such environmental explanations could also
potentially account for the connection between low birth weight, height,
and adult educational and economic attainment. Poverty and stress, if
they spanned significant portions of the prenatal and postnatal periods,
could account for low-birth-weight status (as we pointed out in the last
chapter), as well as for height and adult class status. This is perhaps a
less likely scenario, though, since the evidence presenting a biological
explanation for this three-part model used identical twins, which likely
factors out most of the environmental variation that would be necessary
for such an account to be complete.

INCOME, ENVIRONMENT, AND CHANCES FOR ADULT
SUCCESS: NONBIOLOGICAL CAUSATION

There is a great deal of evidence connecting poverty in childhood to
low educational attainment. As we briefly mentioned earlier, poverty—
like low birth weight—is strongly associated with cognitive ability and
behavioral problems, both of which can have obvious effects on educational and economic attainment.[38] Judith Smith and her colleagues found
that, between the ages of three and eight, relatively small increases in

income can lead to substantial changes in children's intellectual skills. A one-unit increase in the ratio of a family's income to its needs was associated with a 3.0- to 3.7-point increase in measures of verbal and math ability in this study.[39] At young ages, children in poverty are also much more likely than nonpoor children to exhibit behavioral problems in the forms of aggression, tantrums, anxiety, and moodiness. At older ages, after entrance into school, children in poverty begin to show further disorders in the forms of learning and attention problems and school disengagement.[40] Of course, these income differences were not randomly assigned.

But income by itself can have no direct effect on a child's developing brain, and therefore we must consider mediating mechanisms. Money— materially speaking—is only paper, so income differences must take effect via the resources that come with money. More often than not, researchers argue that it is the child's environment that plays this mediating role connecting income to well-being and outcomes.[41] That is, they often assume that income affects social and material circumstances, which in turn affect well-being or outcomes. In the case of cognitive ability, economic limitations may hinder poor parents from providing the intellectually stimulating facilities necessary for proper development. Several studies have found that poor homes have fewer toys and books, implying that low-income children perhaps have fewer opportunities to learn and develop academic skills.[42] Additionally, low-income children often receive lower-quality child care or preschool education, generally offering fewer positive interactions between the child and the caregiver and less opportunity for play.[43] Such negative environmental characteristics can hinder both intellectual and social or behavioral development. Economic limitations may also subject poor parents to chronic stress, which in turn may lead to poor parenting behavior. Research suggests that parents living in poverty are more likely than parents in better conditions to display punitive behaviors—such as shouting, yelling, slapping—and less likely to display love and warmth through behaviors like cuddling and hugging.[44] A great deal of evidence has connected such parenting practices to low IQ scores and to behavioral disorders.[45]

Poverty has also been linked to several health conditions. Although low birth weight is by far the largest health concern for children born into poverty, such children also often lag nonpoor children in growth, receipt of recommended health care, and timeliness of immunizations.[46] At older ages, poverty is further associated with elevated risks for asthma, lower respiratory disease, and lead poisoning.[47] Such health complications are often the result of a deleterious environment. For instance, asthma and lead poisoning both have well-documented connections to environmental factors (i.e., air quality and the use of lead-based paint in the home).[48] In other cases, health complications among poor children can be connected to a lack of adequate health care. Researchers generally agree that one of the main reasons that poor children exhibit higher rates of illness is that they are less likely to have early intervention. Evidence has shown that only 56 percent of poor children with Medicaid coverage received routine care in physicians' offices, versus 82 percent of children living above the poverty line.[49]

While each of these examples of economic causation is entirely plausible, it could also be argued that none of them is entirely reliable in that none completely rules out the possibility of noneconomic causation. Each of the pathways outlined above could be reversed and remain about equally plausible. For instance, rather than a lack of income leading to poor parenting practices and such parental characteristics then leading to a child's low educational attainment, it could alternatively be that parental characteristics are leading to low income as well as to a child's low educational attainment. Suppose a parent is particularly short-tempered. We could imagine this tendency making it hard for this parent to keep a job, while also having negative consequences for his or her child's development. In this case, noneconomic characteristics are leading to economic circumstances, not the other way around. We may be dealing here with a case of reverse causation: because certain noneconomic characteristics tend to be accompanied by certain economic characteristics, it can be difficult to tell whether income is leading to noneconomic characteristics (like temperament and parenting techniques) or such noneconomic characteristics are leading to income level.

This potential role of noneconomic characteristics in children's well-being and outcomes has been most thoroughly explored by Susan Mayer in her book *What Money Can't Buy: Family Income and Children's Life Chances.*[50] In this study, Mayer attempts to untangle the effects of parental income from parental characteristics step-by-step. To begin with, she compares the effects of different sources of income on children's outcomes. Parents may get money from several different sources— earnings, government transfers, and so forth—and Mayer assumes that each of these different sources of income is associated with parental characteristics to differing degrees. For instance, earnings and welfare payments are likely oppositely associated with education. Focusing on the effects of unearned income on kids' outcomes, Mayer compares the effects of parents' welfare receipts (which are strongly associated with parental characteristics) to other forms of unearned income (which are so diverse as to be only weakly associated with parental characteristics). If income helps children, a dollar from welfare should be as valuable as a dollar from other sources of unearned income. Such a uniform effect does not appear to be the case, however. The effect of other, non-welfare forms of unearned income is smaller than the effect of total income. Thus, it seems that parental characteristics may be significantly bound up in the effects of income.

To further sort out the effects of income and parental characteristics, Mayer takes advantage of the role of temporal ordering in causality. For a factor to cause an outcome, the factor must generally occur temporally prior to that outcome. Any statistical effect of a supposedly causal factor that is found after the outcome has already taken place cannot possibly be playing a causal role in the outcome. Using such logic, Mayer compares the effects of parental income before an event, like a teenager having a baby or dropping out of high school, with the effect of parental income after the event. If the effect of income after the event is sizable, it may be assumed that there are significant underlying factors in this measure. Mayer does indeed find that "post-event income" is a strong predictor of children's outcomes, and argues that income effects on children's outcomes may be acting simply as a proxy for unmeasured parental traits.

Mayer further tests some of the more popular theories about income and parental traits, first, by comparing how rich and poor parents spend their money. Mayer finds that high-income parents tend to spend their excess income buying larger homes and cars and eating out more often— all of which likely have little effect on children's outcomes. (However, this is questionable since things like a large house may send subtle messages to children about values and status.) In contrast, the material items widely believed to facilitate child development and improve outcomes, such as books and visits to a museum, Mayer finds are only weakly related to income. So rich and poor children appear about equally likely to have the amenities considered important to outcomes. Mayer suggests this is likely because these items cost so little that their distribution depends more on parental tastes than actual income.

Next, Mayer considers the effect of income on parents' psychological well-being, testing the hypothesis that poverty leads to bad parenting via stress. Mayer finds very little support, though, for this hypothesis and documents only a weak relationship between parents' income and how they interact with their children. Thus, income also appears to have little appreciable influence on children's outcomes through its effects on parents' psychological well-being or parenting practices.

Mayer's book has received a great deal of attention and casts serious doubt on much of the prior research documenting the importance of income on kid's outcomes. Mayer is quick to note, however, that her findings are meaningful only once children's basic material needs are satisfied. In other words, she interprets her results to mean that, once a certain income threshold is passed, characteristics of the parents become more important than anything additional money can buy. It should be noted, though, that even in this sophisticated work we encounter potential sources of bias. Specifically, some of Mayer's techniques may bias income effects in the opposite direction from traditional analysis—that is, toward no effect. When considering the comparison of different sources of parental income, we must wonder what is included in the category of "parents' other unearned income." Mayer works with the same set of data (the PSID) that we use in this book, and based on our knowledge of them, Mayer is referring to inheritance, profit from investments, gifts, and other windfalls. These sources of income are associated with very atypical events and therefore may be related to other changes, such as death of a relative, which may have negative impacts on children. The one source of income here that would seem the most unaffected by other relevant changes—investment income—is really moot for the poor since they get almost none of their income from this source. This potential role of wealth also means that, if income is nonlinear in its effects (as Mayer herself argues when saying that her results are only meaningful when basic needs are satisfied), the income changes that are reflected in the effects of "parents' other unearned income" are largely among the already well-off, where they should matter less anyway.

Additionally, Mayer's comparison of the effects of income before and after an event, as well as her analyses of parents' spending habits and stress levels, could be interpreted as support for traditional arguments of economic causation. The impact of parental income that is captured by post-event income could actually be the effect of pre-event income on both the child's outcome and on post-event parental income. That is, parental income could at time one cause both the event (say, a teenager dropping out of school) and income at time two. This is statistically indistinguishable from Mayer's interpretation of spuriousness. To the extent that parental income is causing *both* the event and future parental income, then it appears spurious and insignificant to Mayer when it is really causal.

INTERACTING RISK FACTORS

Separating out the effects of income, environment, and biology is indeed quite complicated, and in reality, none of these factors acts in isolation. Rather, they act together, often interacting with and depending on one another over the life course and across generations. As we documented in chapter 3, a family tendency toward low birth weight may be exacerbated when parents live in poverty. Any one of multiple scenarios could be behind this relationship. If the mother does not get adequate or timely prenatal care or if neighborhood or employment situations stop her from practicing healthy habits, the likelihood that the present tendency toward low birth weight will express itself through either a premature birth or through growth retardation is heightened. Such interactions between birth weight and environment could continue on through infancy and childhood. When a child is born in poor health because of prematurity and/or low birth weight, the stress and strain that poor parents already feel may be significantly heightened. The prospect of raising such a vulnerable child in a dangerous neighborhood with few resources may then depress many parents. The fact that a sick child is less responsive and animated than other children may even further depress parents, making them feel as though they are not being good parents or as though there is little they can offer their child. Such parents, feeling increasingly overwhelmed, may respond by not interacting with their child as frequently or in as positive a manner as other parents. This pattern will only increase the lack of responsiveness in the child, so that, even when these parents make a large effort to engage their baby, they will not meet with encouragement. Such environmental factors can combine and continue to interact with the child's biological tendency toward slow development, and by the time the child is two or three years old she may be significantly behind in language and cognitive development.[51]

A great deal of empirical evidence points toward such biosocial interactions in the development of low-birth-weight and premature infants. Poverty has been shown to interact with low birth weight to produce particularly deleterious outcomes for LBW children.[52] One study found that, while low income doubled the odds of school failure for normal-birth-weight children, it more than tripled the odds for low-birth-weight children.[53] Environmental factors and intellectual stimulation have also been linked to the life chances of biologically at-risk children.[54] For instance, one study considering children at risk for mental retardation found that high levels of participation in programs that provide intellectual stimulation reduced rates of subnormal IQ. According to this study, only approximately 2 percent of children with high participation levels in intervention programs were in the mentally retarded range, while 13 percent of those with low participation levels fell into this range.[55] Other studies have focused primarily on the home environment, finding that characteristics such as cigarette smoking, number of children, and mother-child interaction play crucial roles in the development of low-birth-weight children.[56] One study found that for LBW children (particularly those born to young mothers) coresidence with the grandmother increased the child's cognitive and mental abilities.[57] Several studies have also shown relationships between income and home environment, thus supporting the argument that home environment mediates the relationship between low birth weight and income.[58] Overall, there is a great deal of evidence pointing to the importance of environment in the effects of biological risk factors. However, as is to be expected in cases of biosocial interactions, the severity of biological risk may affect the salience of environmental factors. For example, there is evidence suggesting that environment has much less of an effect on the development of very-low-birth-weight infants weighing less than 1,500 grams than on that of low-birth-weight infants weighing more than 1,500 grams.[59]

So far, we have documented the inheritance of low birth weight across generations. To the extent that low birth weight may be concentrated within particular families, certain developmental disadvantage may also be concentrated in these families. As the above discussion suggests, environmental risk may also be inherited across generations. So, to the extent that poverty is concentrated within particular families, similar developmental disadvantage may be concentrated in these families. And, to the degree that low birth weight and poverty can be found in the same families across generations, we may find groups at particularly high risk for developmental disadvantage. In the following analyses we are concerned with how these various factors may combine and translate into reduced chances for socioeconomic success for low-birth-weight individuals. To the degree that we find a strong effect of low birth weight in predicting an individual's chances of socioeconomic success, we may uncover an important effect of biological risk in the intergenerational inheritance of poverty. That is, if the inheritance of low birth weight is accompanied by reduced chances of socioeconomic success, we may be able to explain the concentration of low birth weight in lower socioeconomic strata and the transmission of low income across generations. In addition, to the degree that we find that low birth weight determines life chances, we may also document the importance of health as a causal variable in socioeconomic status.

RESEARCH QUESTIONS AND APPROACH

To address these issues, we examine life chances both figuratively (in terms of socioeconomic opportunities and success) and literally (in terms of infant survival). We first examine the effect of low birth weight and childhood environment (along with a number of related factors) on an individual's chances of completing high school by the end of the 19th year of life (figurative life chances). Timely graduation is a substantively important variable with respect to life chances because those who graduate "late" are more likely to receive a high school equivalency degree (GED), which is associated with poorer economic outcomes and lower chances of attending a four-year college.[60] In order to ensure, though, that the results of this analysis are not unique to the single outcome of timely graduation, we further test three additional educational measures: being held back a grade, being enrolled in special education, and being classified as learning disabled. Most prior evidence suggests that poverty in early childhood has a much stronger effect on educational attainment than does poverty later in life.[61] So when considering environment in the following analyses, we examine socioeconomic conditions in the first five years of life. Putting these measurements together with our knowledge of children's low-birth-weight status, we address the following questions: Does low birth weight status affect an individual's chances of educational achievement, independently of income and other socioeconomic conditions during early childhood? And does the effect of low-birth-weight status on educational achievement depend on income during early childhood?

Statistical techniques in the following analyses approximate those used in the previous chapter. That is, we first compare outcomes across families and then, to control for selection bias, we compare outcomes between siblings. This approach is illustrated graphically in Figure 4.1.

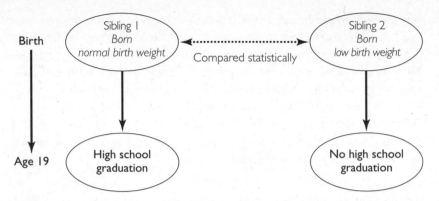

Figure 4.1. Sibling fixed-effects model, part II

Thus in the following analysis, as was also the case in chapter 3, differences in income between sibling cases represent changes in a family's income between two points in time. These differences in sibling's birth weights and early childhood income are then used to predict their respective likelihoods of graduating from high school by age 19.

THE LINGERING IMPLICATIONS OF LOW BIRTH WEIGHT

In the first part of our analysis of the consequences of birth weight, we focus on whether low birth weight children are any less likely to graduate high school in a timely fashion, that is, by their 19th birthday. To best estimate the "true" effects of low birth weight on educational attainment, we rely on both between-family comparison models and sibling, within-family comparison models. Each kind of model informs us in a different way. Our between-family models examine the determinants of timely high school graduation based on a large sample of children. Our within-family focus more narrowly on differences between siblings within families. This latter type of model may be deemed more effective at teasing out pure effects of the variable of interest—in our case, low-birth-weight status—but this approach is more demanding of the data. We will see shortly how these demands may limit the inferences we would wish to draw from the data.

The first bar in Figure 4.2 shows that, when comparing across families, low-birth-weight babies are 32 percent less likely to graduate high school in a timely fashion than those who were not born low birth weight. (Please refer to appendix A for details regarding the calculation of changes in probability.) When forming this comparison in the logis-

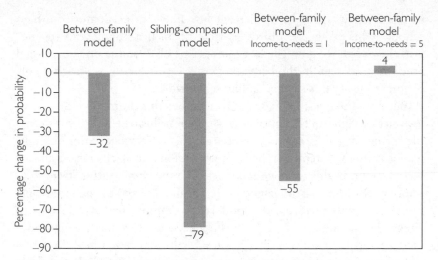

Figure 4.2. The impact of low birth weight on timely high school graduation, using between-family and sibling-comparison models The probability change in column 4 is insignificantly different from zero. See appendix B, Table 4.1, for descriptive statistics associated with these variables; Table 4.3 (columns 1, 2, and 3) for regression coefficients associated with this analysis.

tic models in this figure, we factor out the possibly confounding effects of several variables that we know to bear some relation to a child's educational experience. These include the child's sex, race, parity status (i.e., whether he or she was firstborn); his or her mother's age, marital status, and education at the time of the birth; and the income-to-needs ratio during the first five years of life.

Some would argue that, despite controlling for these confounding variables, we still have not controlled enough. It is again possible that unobserved characteristics of families are at work, giving rise to the educational outcomes we observe. This problem necessitates the use of fixed-effects models, in which many such unobserved attributes of families can be discounted appropriately. If we compare siblings within the same family, we can effectively counter this criticism to the extent that changes in unobserved variables do not occur within a given family.

To address this possibility, we compare timely high school graduation across siblings, rather than across families. The second bar of Figure 4.2 shows a very large and significant negative coefficient for the low-birth-weight variable in this context. When we control for unobserved variation across families by comparing siblings, we see that the estimated impact of LBW status is substantial. An LBW child is shown in this framework to be 79 percent less likely to graduate from high school by his or her 19th birthday than his or her sibling who was not born low birth weight. The large impact of LBW status on educational attainment as seen in the between-family results, then, is strongly corroborated using this stricter sibling framework.

But now the question arises as to whether this dramatic influence of low birth weight on educational attainment holds true uniformly across the socioeconomic spectrum. To address this refinement of our analysis, we measure the interaction between the income-to-needs ratio and low birth weight. In this way, we can determine the comparative strength of the impact of low birth weight for lower-income versus higher-income families. In other words, the models we employ further allow us to gauge the nuances in the relationship between low birth weight and income and their joint influence on educational outcomes. To assess the possibility of the impact of low birth weight on timely high school graduation varying according to a child's level of economic well-being, we contrast two quite different levels of income—namely the income-to-needs ratios of 1.0 and 5.0. The poverty threshold for a family of four in 2001 was $18,104. These two ratios would then imply family-of-four incomes of $18,104 and $90,520, respectively—that is, a family straddling the poverty line versus one that is, by most people's standards, well-off.

For purposes of gleaning the effect of this interaction on high school graduation, we rely on our between-family analysis. Although family fixed-effects modeling is a powerful technique, it is important to mention once again that in this framework changes in income are noted only across a given family's reproductive careers. That is, we take note of changes in income that, for example, might have occurred between the birth of a woman's first and second child. Such changes are considerably smaller, on average, than the variation we observe in income across families. Put another way, the typical range of year-to-year income variations in any one family pales in comparison to the range of income differences among all families on a national basis. As a consequence, the impact of such small changes in income for individual families is very difficult to detect (and we do not detect a significant income effect in this framework, either alone or contingent on sibling birth weight differences). That said, it should in no way be inferred from an insignificant income coefficient that income has no bearing on a child's educational attainment. Rather, by the very nature of our statistical framework—in this case, the fixed-effects approach—the effects of income are simply not sensitive enough to the small changes in income we observe within families to enable us to obtain significant results.

In the last two bars of Figure 4.2, we use the across-family approach to document the impact of being born low birth weight on timely high school graduation for children of families at these very different income levels. Low-birth-weight status matters tremendously for children born at the poverty line. A low birth weight child whose family's income-to-needs ratio is 1.0 is 55 percent less likely to graduate high school by his or her 19th birthday than a non-low-birth-weight child born at the poverty line. Among children born into families who are well-off (with an income-to-needs ratio of 5.0) the story is quite different: an LBW child born into these economic circumstances has a probability of graduating high school in a timely fashion virtually identical to (a trivial 4 percent greater than) that of a non-LBW child.

These results suggest that, if we took two siblings at the poverty level who were similar in all *observable* ways that are represented in the survey, except for their birth weight status, a low-birth-weight child would be much less likely to succeed in educational terms than a non-low-birth-weight child. Two siblings—one low birth weight, one not—who were relatively well-off, in contrast, would not fare differently, however.

In these cross-family models, it appears that biology and society interact very significantly, such that low birth weight matters much more when a child is at socioeconomic risk. We learn that a high income appears to counteract or serve as a buffer for the potentially deleterious effects of low birth weight on high school graduation. Birth weight appears to have a striking effect on one's education prospects, but only among children who do not have the good fortune to be born into economically successful families.

LOW BIRTH WEIGHT AND OTHER EDUCATIONAL OUTCOMES

To be sure that these large effects of low birth weight are robust—that is, that they are found beyond the single case of timely high school graduation—we repeat the above models with different educational outcome measures. More specifically, we examine whether low birth weight is an important predictor of an individual having to repeat a grade, being placed in special education, or being classified as learning disabled.[62] Examining only the single measure of timely high school graduation could be problematic. For instance, the above evidence showing that low-birth-weight children are graduating later than normal-birth-weight

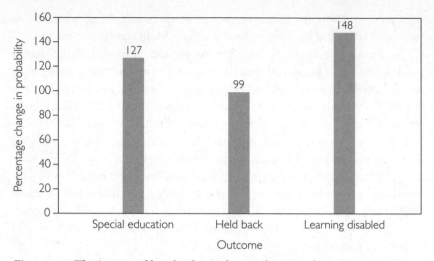

Figure 4.3. The impact of low birth weight on educational attainment, using between-family models. See appendix B, Table 4.4 (columns 1, 3, and 5), for regression coefficients associated with this analysis.

children could result not from low-birth-weight children having more educational problems than normal-birth-weight children but from a tendency for low-birth-weight children to begin school later. Since LBW children are more likely than non-LBW children to suffer from prematurity and early health problems, it may be more likely that parents delay LBW children's entrance into kindergarten, thus causing low-birth-weight children to graduate later than their normal-birth-weight counterparts even if their educational progress is seamless from kindergarten on. In this case, the above results would not really represent the ongoing consequences of birth weight—as we have suggested—but would rather be an indirect reflection of an early condition associated with low birth weight. To be sure that such that such an alternative scenario is not taking place, we consider these alterative indicators of educational attainment.

Figure 4.3 shows that, in our between-family models, being born low birth weight significantly increases the chances that a child will be enrolled in special education, held back a grade, or classified as learning disabled. Indeed, a child who was born low birth weight has a 127 percent higher chance of being enrolled in special education than a child born in a normal weight range, a 99 percent higher chance of being held back a grade, and a 148 percent higher chance of being classified as learning disabled. It appears that low birth weight matters for several educational outcomes beyond timely high school graduation and that the later graduation dates of low-birth-weight children documented above cannot be attributed entirely to delayed entrance into kindergarten. That is, low-birth-weight status appears to be shaping children's educational progress in multiple ways over several years.

In our within-family comparisons in this analysis, birth weight status does not have a significant effect on one's chances of being enrolled in special education, being held back a grade, or being classified as learning disabled.[63] We cannot really interpret this result as meaning that birth weight has no bearing on educational progress, however, because our within-family comparisons are very limited in this analysis. As already pointed out, all our within-family models are limited to those families in which the siblings are discordant on birth weight and on the outcome measure. So in our analysis of high school graduation, for instance, our sample was restricted to families in which one sibling was low birth weight and the other sibling was normal birth weight, and one sibling graduated "on time" while the other sibling did not. This within-family variation is necessary so that we actually have differences to compare in the within-family models.

In this analysis of special education, grade repetition, and learning disability, this requirement of within-family models proves quite limiting. Being enrolled in a special education program, repeating a grade, and being classified as learning disabled are relatively rare events. Indeed, in our sample (which has a higher-than-average number of children at high risk for these outcomes because of poverty status) only 5.5 percent of children had been treated as learning disabled, and a similarly small amount had been in special education (5.4 percent). A somewhat larger proportion had repeated a grade at some point in their educational careers (10.2 percent). The low rates for these outcomes mean that, once we limit our sample to those families with children of different birth weights and only one child with the relevant outcome, its size is so small that drawing substantive conclusions is difficult. In the case of our special education analysis, for instance, the size of our sample drops from 1,057 to 106 when we switch to within-family comparisons.[64] Consequently, we are dealing with such a small group of families in our within-family comparisons that we cannot be confident that these results would apply to families outside this group. We can note, though, that the estimates of low birth weight's effects in our within-family models (while statistically insignificant) do operate in the same direction as the estimates in our between-family comparisons. That is, in these models our low-birth-weight estimates are positively related to being held back a grade, being classified as learning disabled, and being enrolled in special education. Our evidence does consistently suggest that low birth weight has deleterious consequences on education, even if we must treat some of these suggestions as more reliable than others.

A POUND OF FLESH OR JUST PROXY?
BIRTH WEIGHT AND INFANT MORTALITY

The second portion of this analysis works backward in time from age 19 to age 1. Specifically, we examine how birth weight affects the risk of infant mortality for twin siblings. As mentioned previously, low birth weight is often used as a stand-in for a variety of health problems; most notably, it can reflect preterm delivery or can result from intrauterine growth retardation (i.e., smallness for gestational age). In fact, throughout this text, we have often used prematurity and low birth weight interchangeably since much of the literature does not distinguish between these two etiologies. Furthermore, within these two rather broad categories, there may be a large degree of heterogeneity in both the social (distal) and biological (proximal) causes and consequences of low birth weight. Even the sibling comparisons shown above cannot distinguish when a pound of flesh (i.e., birth weight) really matters from when it is acting as a proxy for overall pregnancy and perinatal health conditions. For example, we do not distinguish between premature births and small-for-gestational-age infants—let alone make further medical distinctions within these broad risk categories (because such information is not available in our main data set, the PSID). We also cannot account for other unobserved differences (social or biological) between one pregnancy and another that may underlie the association we observe between birth weight and the children's outcomes. Finally, since siblings share on average only 50 percent of their genes, we do not know whether sibling birth weight differences are a result of innate genetic differences that may in turn be causally implicated in the educational attainment results as well.

The following portion of the analysis attempts to address these lacunae. We examine twin births from the Matched Multiple Birth Database, which includes all recorded multiple births in the United States between 1995 and 1997.[65] For several reasons we restrict our analysis to twin pairs who were both born alive. First, twins shared the same pregnancy, so if, for example, the mother smoked or drank during her pregnancy, this presumably affected both twins. If she was under a lot of social stress due to a bad marriage, job, financial pressures, or other factors, this also affected both twins. While there are environmental differences within the womb (such as the position of each fetus), they are largely unrelated to environmental conditions outside the womb. Second, examining twins removes confusion between prematurity and growth retardation. While most twins do not go to the full, 40-week gestation that is the norm for singleton births (and many do not make the 37-week cutoff for "maturity" status), both twins are—very atypical circumstances aside—born at the same time plus or minus a matter of minutes or hours. Thus, birth weight differences between twins are not likely to be acting as a proxy for gestational age (though they may be conditional on maturity). Finally, separating out the effect of birth weight differences for fraternal twins from that for identical twins gives us some purchase on the role of birth weight as a proxy for the infant's genetic "robustness." If all our twin sets were fraternal, we could not be sure whether weight differences were acting as stand-ins for general health, potential brain development, or some other genotypic difference that mattered for long-term life chances. However, by isolating the effects of birth weight differences among identical twin sets, we can purge our estimates of underlying genetic differences. In other words, while birth weight differences between fraternal twins may still reflect differences in the health and well-being of the fetus-turned-infant, birth weight differences between identical twins are a seemingly random event. In this we are following much the same approach that Jere Behrman and Mark Rosenzweig used in the study of birth weight and adult height and income described earlier in this chapter.

However, their data set has *only* identical twins, so a question remains: are the effects of birth weight differences among identical twins overstated when generalized to the entire population? Because our data set contains both identical and fraternal twins, we can begin to address this issue. Imagine that each child in the world has a genetically "optimal" birth weight. For one child this may be six pounds and for another it may be seven pounds. Let us further imagine that within some acceptable range each child attained this weight. For child 1, six pounds represents full development. For child 2, the extra pound of flesh really reflects not more consequential fetal development but rather a genetic tendency. In this case, there may be no real effect of that pound difference in birth weight—each child is at his or her ideal weight. However, compare this to the situation of identical twins, where we know that—by definition—the ideal birth weight for each is the same. We already know that there are nutrient competition and space limitations in the womb such that neither twin will likely reach his or her genetically "ideal" weight. For example, in our PSID sample of singleton births, the mean birth weight is 7.5 pounds. Compare that with the mean birth weight for the twin sample of 5.25 pounds.[66]

Fraternal twin differences in weight are due not only to the competition between the fetuses for resources and the random event of who is in better position vis-à-vis the placenta but also to those genetically inherent differences in bulkiness we discussed above. Contrast this with identical twins. The difference in the weight of identical twins necessarily means that one was more deprived than the other. That is, the only source of weight difference is the random event of who got the lucky seat in the womb. Let us now imagine a scenario in which the impact of birth weight differences on the twin-specific risk for death between identical twins is stronger than that for fraternal twins. This would lead us to the conclusion that birth weight differences among twins resulting from sibling rivalry for nutrients are really much more salient than those resulting from underlying genetic differences. In other words, nutritional deprivation is really what matters, and therefore it would be dangerous to generalize from the identical twin (or the fraternal twin) population to all babies, since we know that this nutritional risk is much greater on average among the twin sets. It is precisely this possibility that Behrman and Rosenzweig cannot rule out. Generalizing in this case would translate to sounding the alarms for that one-pound difference between child 1 and child 2 when it really does not matter since they are each at their genetically ideal weight.

However, if the effect of birth weight differences turns out to be stronger for fraternal twins than for identical twins, our estimates of birth weight difference in the population as a whole (such as those that we found in educational outcomes) may be biased upward. This is because birth weight differences in the population as a whole (and in the fraternal twin sample) reflect underlying genetic differences as well as weight/nutrition/development differences in utero. Ideally, then, this database of multiple births would have followed its subjects up through age 19, so we could reproduce the findings from the PSID singleton sample. Of course, having been born between 1995 and 1997, these twin sets have no educational record to speak of. Instead, we use infant mortality as our outcome, with the assumption that the same risks that would predict infant death also would predict poor socioeconomic outcomes among the survivors.[67]

To bolster this assumption, we break down the analysis of infant mortality into neonatal and postneonatal categories. Neonatal mortality—death in the first 30 days of life—is usually reflective of some serious underlying medical problem, often congenital in nature. Postneonatal mortality (death during days 31 to 365) is less likely to be the result of serious perinatal complications and is more sensitive to general developmental issues. Examining the differences in the effects of birth weight by zygosity on these two mortality time frames opens a window for understanding what types of bias emerge or disappear as we move farther from the starting gate of life. For example, if for neonatal mortality the effects of birth weight are the same for fraternal and identical twins but for postneonatal mortality birth weight seems to matter only for fraternal twins, this suggests that after an initial "weeding out" process, any lingering effects of birth weight really reflect underlying genetic differences. This possibility would suggest that our results for birth weight's impact on education by age 19 are largely reflecting underlying differences among the children and do not accurately capture the effects of poundage per se. However, the opposite dynamic could hold. That is, envision the scenario in which the effect of birth weight is more severe for fraternal twins in the first stage of life (neonatal mortality) but then, as we progress outward from the starting gate, equalizes for fraternal and identical twins. This would suggest that early in life—during that weeding-out process—birth weight may often be acting as a proxy for congenital differences but any longer-term consequences are related to the weight itself. Of course, our analysis could show that, as we move from the starting gate, the effects diminish entirely for both groups.

All of these machinations are contingent on several assumptions. First and most important, we can distinguish between fraternal and identical twin sets. Since our data come from national natality and death records, they contain no recorded zygosity indicator. However, given the overall prevalence of fraternal and identical twins in the population, we can impute differences between fraternal and identical twin sets. Genetically identical, or monozygotic, twins occur in about 3.5 per 1,000 births (or 1 in 285 births). This rate is generally assumed to be universal and random, since it holds constant across race, ethnicity, and geography.[68] However, one's chances of having identical twins does increase at younger and older ages, so some have hypothesized that the likelihood of identical twins may be dependent on hormonal imbalances seen at these ages (although the factors affecting identical twinning are generally very poorly understood).[69]

The occurrence of fraternal, or dizygotic, twins, in contrast, is not so universal or random and varies systematically by several factors. For instance, there is sizable variation in rates of fraternal twins across nations. Japan has a very low fraternal twin rate, only about 6 per 1,000 births (or 1 in 166), while Nigeria has a strikingly high 45 per 1,000 births (or 1 in 22). The United States lies in between these two countries with about 11 of 1,000 births being fraternal twins (or 1 in 90).[70] Further, as we might expect based on such variations, twin rates also vary significantly by race and ethnicity. White rates of twin births are often significantly lower (1 in 69 births) than black rates (1 in 40, although this difference is decreasing in the United States with the increased use of infertility treatments among whites). However, rates of fraternal twin births among Asian groups tend to be even lower than those for white groups. For individuals of Japanese descent about 1 in 150 births are twins, while for those of Chinese descent about 1 in 250 births are twins.[71]

The likelihood that a woman will give birth to fraternal twins varies by several additional factors. For instance, one's chances of having fraternal twins increase with one's height and weight, with younger age at first menstruation, and with a shorter menstrual cycle.[72] One of the most important recent factors affecting the chances of twin births, however, is a marked increase in the use of infertility treatments, particularly among older, middle-class, and white women. Largely because of these treatments, sizable shifts are occurring in the epidemiology of multiple births. Overall, the number of twins in the United States increased from 90,118 to 104,137 in the short time period from 1989 to 1997.[73] Most of this increase appears to have resulted from an increase in the rates of twin births among older women—that is, one of the groups more likely to use infertility treatments. Between 1980 and 1997 the twin birth rate rose 63 percent for women aged 40 to 44 and rose 1,000 percent for women 45 to 49 years old. Indeed, there were more twins born to women aged 45 to 49 in the single year of 1997 than during the entire decade of the 1980s.[74] These changes in rates of twin births, furthermore, have almost eliminated the traditional difference in twin rates between whites and black in the United States. Because white women are more likely than black women to delay childbearing and to seek fertility treatments, white rates of twins are quickly approaching black rates. In 1997, 28.8 of 1,000 births to white women were twins, while 30.0 of 1,000 births to black women were twins.[75] (We do not find, however, significant maternal race or education differences in the analysis we present below.)

In order to deduce zygosity, we must recall that all mixed-sex twin sets are by definition fraternal. And given the proportions of identical twins and fraternal twins in the population, we know that approximately half of the same-sex twin sets are fraternal and half are identical (this is known as Weinberg's rule). Given this, the effect of birth weight in the same-sex sample is really an average of the effect of birth weight among fraternal twins and that among identical twins. This assumes that the effect of birth weight is not conditional on gender differences, of course. Otherwise, we could be misinterpreting what were really gender differences as zygosity differences. Our results show that this is a valid assumption, since in the mixed-sex sample the effect of birth weight does not appear to vary by gender; further, when we break out the same-sex sample into all-boy and all-girl subsets, we find the effect of birth weight to be identical. The inferred results for "identicals" also depend on the fact that the probability of death is the same for both identical and fraternal twins. Since we are using only twin pairs in which one died in the relevant time frame and one did not, this is true by definition. That is, the average probability of death for all groups (and in fact, for every twin set) is 50 percent. Also, our approach depends on the fact that the overall weight and weight differences are the same for fraternal and identical twin sets. There would be reason for concern if the same-sex and opposite-sex twins demonstrated vastly different mean weights or weight discordancies, as well. Our analysis shows this not to be the case, however.

There are other considerations as well. There could be unaccounted-for environmental factors associated with zygosity that are confounding the effects of birth weight differences on infant mortality. All fraternal twins are dichorionic—meaning that they each have their own placenta. However, some identical twins (an estimated 64 to 85 percent of white twins) are monochorionic—they share a placenta. The remaining portion of identical twins that are not monochorionic are, like fraternal twins, dichorionic.[76] Sharing a placenta has been shown to significantly increase the risk of adverse outcomes in twin pregnancies. Because twins in one placenta will be connected to one another via that placenta, the tendency for unequal sharing and for growth discordance is significantly increased for monochorionic twins as compared to dichorionic.[77] Thus, a smaller, genetically identical twin may face increased health risk because of chorionicity, while no fraternal twins will face such increased risk. The issue of monochorionic and dichorionic twins may also confound our ability to accurately estimate the effects of birth weight on mortality by zygosity. In other words, the importance of birth weight differences for identical twins might be contingent on chorionicity.[78] However, unless chorionicity is assessed by an ultrasound in the first trimester or early in the second trimester of a pregnancy, it can be very difficult to measure; thus it is generally not recorded in large data sets such as ours.[79]

Finally, this approach depends on the fact that birth weight differences for all twins, both identical and fraternal, are generalizable to the larger population in some reasonable way. This issue is raised by data documenting higher rates of adverse birth outcomes for twins than for singleton births. While twins make up only about 2 to 2.5 percent of births, they are responsible for 15.8 percent of cases of very low birth weight, 13.7 percent of low-birth-weight cases, and 8.4 percent infant deaths.[80] Further, according to one study, intrauterine growth retardation is much higher among twins (42 percent) than among singleton births (8 percent).[81] We have already seen that the mean weight for the twins is lower by over two pounds. What's more, the average weight difference for twin pairs is larger as a percentage of weight than for sibling pairs. Among the PSID singleton siblings, the average weight difference at birth is 0.5 pound, among the twins 0.61 pound. Expressed as a percentage of total weight this difference is even greater due to the twins' lower weights. This difference matters, however, only if the effects of birth weight are nonlinear or have a series of critical break points. We tested for these possibilities, and they do not appear to hold forth in our data (though the effects of additional pounds may taper off at *very* high birth weights, which are underrepresented among twins).

Figure 4.4 shows the results of our analysis of infant mortality among twins. Overall, a twin who is a pound lighter than his or her sibling is about 19 percent more likely to die in the first year of life. When we separate same-sex from opposite-sex pairs, we find that the effect for same-sex pairs is weaker than for opposite-sex pairs. Following Weinberg's rule, we know that the coefficient for same-sex twins is an average of that for fraternal and identical twins. And we know that the mixed-sex sample is all fraternal. Since we also find no significant gender differences in the effects of birth weight in the mixed-sex pairs or when we split the same-sex sample into boys and girls (see appendix B, Table 4.7), we can be confident that the difference in the effect of birth

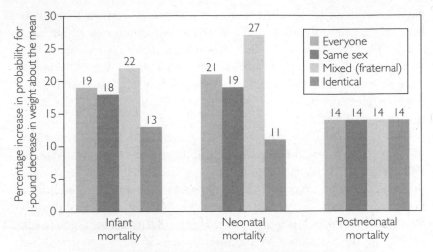

Figure 4.4. The impact of a one-pound increase in birth weight on three measures of infant mortality, using twin-comparison models. See appendix B, Table 4.5, for descriptive statistics associated with these variables; Table 4.6 for regression coefficients associated with infant mortality analysis; Table 4.7 for regression coefficients associated with neonatal mortality analysis; Table 4.8 for regression coefficients associated with postneonatal mortality analysis.

weight among same-sex and opposite-sex twin sets is a result of zygosity differences. With this in mind, the last of the four bars in Figure 4.4 shows the inferred effect of a pound of weight for the identical-twin subsample. While the effect for "fraternals" is such that a twin who is a pound lighter than its sibling is 22 percent more likely to die in the first year of life, the inferred effect for identicals suggests that one less pound of weight increases the risks of death by 13 percent. These results indicate that chorionicity issues are probably overshadowed by the fact that, among fraternals, birth weight may be acting as a proxy for other underlying congenital health conditions, which leads to the excess strength of the estimate for this group as compared to that for the identical twin subset.

In order to better understand the pattern of effects here, we separate this analysis into neonatal and postneonatal time frames. In the middle set of bars in Figure 4.4, we see that, in predicting death in the first month of life, birth weight differences between the twins matter. However, the effect for fraternal twins is much greater than that we infer for identical twins—a difference that is more pronounced than that for overall infant mortality. A fraternal twin who is one pound heavier than his or her sibling is 27 percent less likely to die in the neonatal period, while an identical twin who is one pound heavier than his or her sibling gets only an 11 percent reduction in the risk of neonatal death. This would seem to indicate—chorionicity issues aside—that to a certain extent birth weight is acting as a proxy for other underlying genetic conditions (which vary between fraternal twins and do not between identical twins) that make their presence strongly felt in the first month of life.

This stands in contrast to the effects presented in the last set of bars in Figure 4.4, where the impact of poundage is the same for fraternal and identical twin sets. In predicting postneonatal mortality (conditional on living past day 30 of life), it appears as though each additional pound results in about a 14 percent decrease in the chance of death—for both identical and fraternal twins. This similarity across zygosity suggests that, after an initial weeding-out process in which genetic differences may be behind birth weight effects, birth *weight* per se does indeed appear to have an impact on life chances after accounting for genes. Extending this logic outward 19 years seems to imply that at least some of the effects we observe on educational progress may be responsive to actual weight increases and are not merely proxies for unobserved genetic or pregnancy-specific differences.

CONCLUSION

These findings document the importance of low birth weight in both short- and long-term outcomes. According to our analysis of timely high school graduation, biology clearly matters in terms of educational and—by extension—economic success. Our analysis of grade retention, special education, and learning disabilities offers some further evidence of the lasting consequences of low birth weight. Based on the last chapter, we also know that the biological conditions of the previous generation play a large role in determining this biology. So it appears that inherited biological conditions are important to one's long-term prospects. But, this cycle does not necessarily imply that biology is the only thing that matters. Income also plays a role in determining how biological conditions affect health at birth and chances for success down the road. According to results from chapter 3, income has beneficial effects for those babies facing biological risk, so that if a child has a low-birth-weight parent, income raises her birth weight by more than half a pound. Results from this chapter also suggest that higher incomes may offset the deleterious effects of low birth weight. We have some evidence to suggest that, as a family's income approaches five times the poverty level, the negative effects of low birth weight on high school graduation are reduced. Across lifetimes and generations, environment interacts with biology, and greater economic resources can counteract biological predispositions.

But what about the causal mechanisms that may be behind these long-term effects of low birth weight? In our twin analysis we could factor out the unobserved heterogeneity that we discussed in chapter 1— that is, genetic differences and many of the unobserved prenatal conditions, like mother's behavior (smoking or drinking) and environment (stress or exposure to toxins) that may affect birth weight. Once such confounding elements were mostly taken care of, we found that weight itself—literal poundage—likely plays a causal role in the implications of size at birth—even holding gestational age constant. We found that, after the initial neonatal period, when underlying factors (genetics or other health conditions) are partially behind birth weight effects, poundage itself becomes important, ultimately playing a large role in who survives their first year of life. This implies that weight at birth likely plays some causal role in the educational outcomes that we documented in this chapter. However, even these effects on mortality may be socially mediated; for example, the higher death rates of lower-weight twins could be due to a fragile-child syndrome, meaning that parents treat and care for the infants differently by weight. Indeed, when we examine cause-of-death data for the postneonatal period among the sets of twins where one survived and one did not, we find that the leading cause of death is sudden infant death syndrome (SIDS, also known as crib death). This little-understood phenomenon may be acting as place holder for proximal causes of death that pathologists and pediatricians do not fully understand and that may be more social in nature (that is, affected by parental behavior). Keeping this in mind, the evidence of specific birth *weight* effects does not imply, of course, that other environmental or social factors do not also play a role in affecting the consequences of poundage. In fact, the further we extend our window out from birth, the more likely it is that social factors will come to bear on outcomes—a possibility implied by our findings that low birth weight seems to matter differently for families at different income levels.

Indeed, in the nontwin sibling comparisons that we use to document effects of birth weight on educational attainment, we are considering changes in specific aspects of a family's condition (i.e., class status, maternal age, etc.) over time, and it is still possible that such specific changes may represent the larger life transitions that can occur between births—from young to old maternal age and among various income levels. There may be significant interactions between the specific biological condition of birth weight and subtle aspects of children's environments (other than income) that determine how much low birth weight matters in the long run. Future researchers may want to explore such biosocial interactions. Along the way, they should also investigate the specific reasons that low-birth-weight children appear to end up disadvantaged educationally when compared to their non-low-birth-weight siblings— is it through health problems, cognitive developmental delays, or some other mechanism with a more social basis, like the fragile child syndrome? The answers to these questions and the documentation of biosocial interactions will only help parents, practitioners, and policy makers to best treat these at-risk children.

CHAPTER 5

Reconsidering Risk

Biosocial Policy Implications

It is a greater work to educate a child . . . than to rule a state.
　　William Ellery Channing

This book has used the case study of low birth weight to paint a picture of how nature and nurture work together—across individual lives and generations—to determine life chances. That is, our results have revealed that biological and social advantage or disadvantage, inherited from previous generations, frequently interact with one another to determine a person's social position. According to our results, a family history of low birth weight significantly increases one's risk of being born low birth weight. But if low-birth-weight parents enjoy a high income, the effect of parental low birth weight diminishes. Similarly, having been born low birth weight oneself significantly hinders educational attainment, and hence long-term economic prospects. But if a low-birth-weight child grows up in a household with a high enough income, the biological effects of low birth weight may begin to recede.

Let us consider two families with histories of low birth weight, one with a high income and one with a low income. Based on our results, the family with a high income will likely be able to use their economic resources to counteract their biological risk profile, and their baby is more likely to be born at a normal birth weight. However, the family with a low income does not have the economic resources to protect their baby from the present biological risk, and our results suggest that this baby has a high probability of being born at a low birth weight. As biology and society present a double advantage and double disadvantage for these two babies, we find the stage set for a repeat of this biosocial disparity in the next generation. Our findings suggest that the normal-birth-weight baby born to the higher-income parents has the biological and social resources to excel in school and, as a young adult, is in a position to have high earnings himself. The low birth weight baby born to the lower-income parents, in contrast, has neither the biological nor the social resources to succeed educationally and, as young adult, may not be in a favorable economic position. As these two babies—now adults—get ready to have their own children, the baby who was born to the higher-income parents was probably economically positioned to protect his child against a biological legacy of low birth weight. But the baby born to the lower-income parents is most likely not in such a favorable position and may not be able to protect his child from the biological risk of low birth weight. Thus, taken as a whole, the results of this book suggest that a family's social and biological resources interact with one another, working to replicate economic and health inequality across generations.

What are the implications of these findings? How can we use the results of this book to improve the life chances of children who are born low birth weight or to prevent low birth weight in the first place? In this chapter, we argue that the most effective way to intervene in the inter-generational cycle of low birth weight and economic disadvantage is to carve out new space in existing social policy for biosocial interactions. That is, we propose that resources be targeted at those populations facing *both* biological and social risk. And we further argue that such attention to the intersection of biology and society must be long term, covering the prenatal period, childhood, and young adulthood.

Before making such proposals, though, we must issue a warning. Discussing the intersection of biology and society in inheritance can lead us into some controversial areas with slippery slopes. Focusing on the con-founding of biological and social risk in a developmental framework (particularly before children are born), we almost inevitably encounter issues of heredity where there is likely a genetic component, and this can raise several concerns. As already discussed, the term *genetic* is often associated with the assumption that a condition is predetermined or natural. Thus, considering a biological risk that likely has a genetic component when discussing social position may lead to the inappropriate assumption that social inequality is inevitable, natural, or just. That is, our attention to biology or genetics in this discussion may be misinterpreted or misused as a justification for unequal opportunities or outcomes.

Even discussing biosocial interactions in an after-birth developmental framework can get quite complicated. Here consequences may be more subtle but potentially equally as troubling. Heightening awareness of biological conditions that are strongly associated with social positions may again in some cases attach seemingly "objective" criteria to the unequal denial of opportunities. For instance, one could argue that increases in the medical and biological evidence around conditions such as attention deficit hyperactivity disorder (ADHD) has served only to more clearly justify decisions to take more poor children out of the general education system, thus exacerbating existing inequalities in learning opportunities. In some cases the suggestions we make about the role of low birth weight in education could be misused in a similar way.

In short, the general, often implicit assumption that biology (and genetics) represents a predetermined, objective, and natural situation may be used inappropriately in many cases to justify policies or situations that are not just. But does this mean that policies addressing the intersection of biological and social risk are in themselves problematic? We would argue no. Like almost any knowledge that matters in the long run, attention to the confounding of biological and social risk in economic and health inequalities can be used for various purposes. If evidence of biological or genetic inheritance is misinterpreted in a reductionist fashion as evidence of a predetermined or unalterable condition, it may indeed be used to deny resources or opportunities and to further inequalities. But if evidence is interpreted more carefully and attention is paid to subtle interactions between biological and social risk, it may alternatively be used to effectively target resources and decrease inequalities. The flip side of the above concerns is the possibility that attention to biosocial risk will be used to prevent poverty and poor health and to intervene in intergenerational cycles that maintain such stratification.

PREVENTION

Our results have highlighted the importance of a biological legacy in a baby's risk of low birth weight. But our results have also shown that economic resources play an important role in whether a biological legacy actually leads to a low-birth-weight birth. As we discussed in chapter 3, if a parent was born low birth weight, for every unit increase in a family's income-to-needs ratio, a baby's birth weight rises by more than half a pound (nine ounces). A crucial part of preventing low birth weight, then, will be targeting resources toward pregnant women, particularly those at biological risk for a low-birth-weight birth.

Many of the social policy programs in the United States—ranging from cash assistance to public medical insurance—determine eligibility and benefit levels with two criteria. First, there are categorical criteria. To be eligible for a given program—say, cash assistance—one must fall within an applicable category. For cash assistance, one must be part of a family with a dependent child. Second, there are also financial criteria. One must not only be a member of an applicable category but also have an income below a particular threshold. Here, social programs generally use needs-based tests to assess whether a categorically qualified family's income is sufficient to meet their needs, and if it is insufficient, they are eligible for benefits of a given level. Working within this general framework, we have two main suggestions for how resources may be targeted toward pregnant women, particularly those at biological risk. First, when it is reasonable and possible, family medical histories should be part of the categorical tests that determine eligibility and benefit levels. For instance, we suggest below that a family history of low birth weight should qualify people for special categories and priority statuses in Medicaid and WIC. Second, we believe that many of the needs-based income tests that determine eligibility and benefit levels should take pregnancies into account. In most cases (such as with the federal poverty line), "need" is determined by the number of people in a household. Building on this, we propose that a pregnancy be considered a "qualifying event" that allows for special calculations. For instance, as is currently the case with Medicaid policy, we would like to see in some cases pregnant women count as two individuals in the determination of a household's size and, hence, needs.[1] This would imply that pregnant women with higher incomes would become eligible for many social programs and that all pregnant women, once eligible for certain programs, would be in a position to receive higher levels of benefits.

In making this proposal that a pregnancy be considered in the determination of a household's size, we again enter some controversial territory—this time with regard to abortion politics and women's reproductive rights. Placing a fetus on par with another member of a household—say an additional child—may be interpreted by some to be a statement about the rights of fetuses, and hence the legality of abortion. Even though we can state up front that we do not intend our suggestion to have any implications for women's reproductive rights, the line between targeting resources toward pregnant women and infringing on women's reproductive rights can, at times, be vague.

Indeed, the position of unborn children and pregnant women in the U.S. welfare system is rather ambiguous in general, and the politics surrounding related programs can at times center more on symbolism and emotion than on substantive needs and resources. For instance, this issue recently led to heated debates over the State Child Health Insurance Program (SCHIP). In 2002 the Bush administration announced its intention to "expand the definition of a child eligible for coverage under the Child Health Insurance Program to begin with conception."[2] While the administration claimed it was simply "trying to expand coverage for prenatal care to women who might not otherwise receive it," reproductive rights advocates disagreed, claiming it was "a backdoor effort to expand legal protection for fetuses and restrict the legal rights of women."[3] We do not deny the possibility that the Bush administration had ulterior motives in making this proposal or that the proposal may pose a significant threat to women's reproductive rights. However, this controversy seems to have more to do with the political framing of and the language attached to this proposal than with the more substantive goals at hand. It is likely that women's rights advocates would not have responded so negatively if the Bush administration's anti-choice position had not previously been stated clearly and if the explicit use of the word *child* in the title of the program did not send an implicit message about the administration's views on what the position of fetuses should be. It seems that the context of this proposal (while no doubt meaningful) is more in question than its goals.

This distinction between substance and context becomes clearer if we contrast this Bush proposal with the case of Medicaid. As we mentioned above, pregnant women are counted as two individuals in the calculation of needs for Medicaid eligibility; thus fetuses are treated as equivalent to other members of a household in this program. Yet we know of no controversy surrounding this aspect of Medicaid. Likely because the wording of the legislation makes no explicit reference to children, this Medicaid proposal did not meet with the same negative reaction as Bush's SCHIP proposal. Thus, it seems that the goal of providing more services to pregnant women is generally not controversial. Further, it seems that giving fetuses an explicit role in the eligibility procedures for a program is not always controversial but rather depends on the political framing of and symbolism surrounding the proposal. For example, it is worth considering how various political constituencies would have reacted had Bush proposed "PWHIP"—the pregnant women's health insurance program—with precisely the same parameters and eligibility requirements as his controversial trial balloon. We imagine the reaction would have been quite different, even welcoming in some of the quarters that have been the most hostile to his current proposal.

Again, here we encounter a situation in which our suggestions could be used for multiple purposes. While our proposal to count fetuses within existing policy frameworks is meant to offer resources to pregnant women in an efficient manner, it may alternatively be misused to justify changes in abortion law. Yet as was the case above, we cannot let this potential misuse or controversy force us to abandon our efforts to prevent low birth weight. The flip side of the possibility that our suggestion will be misinterpreted is the (we hope more likely) possibility that it will allow further resources to reach pregnant women and thus will help prevent low birth weight. In short, while we recognize that our findings and their implications may inadvertently lead us into some grey or controversial areas, we also believe that we should not allow the potential good that can result from these findings or suggestions to be held hostage by the potential for misinterpretation.

Preventive Programs

There are several social policy programs to which our suggestions about biosocial interactions may be applied.

Medicaid.   First, we consider Medicaid, a joint federal-state program that provides health insurance to low-income Americans. Under Medicaid, states have separate insurance programs that allow eligible individuals to obtain health care services from hospitals and providers—state reimbursements to providers of care are then partially matched by the federal government. Medicaid does indeed play a very large role in infant health, providing prenatal care to many low-income women and covering approximately one in three births in the United States.[4]

Eligibility for Medicaid can be rather complex. While certain Medicaid guidelines are set by the federal government, a fair amount of leeway in these guidelines allows for significant variation in eligibility and benefits across states. For instance, within federally defined eligibility boundaries, there are divisions between "mandatory" and "optional" services that allow states a great deal of flexibility in who and what they cover.

The first group of eligibility categories under Medicaid refers to those defined as "categorically needy." This group is "mandatory," meaning that all states must provide coverage to everyone within these categories. As of 2002, pregnant women whose family income is below 133 percent of the federal poverty line fall into this group because all states are required to provide coverage to these women.[5] This standard means that single pregnant women in any state can qualify for prenatal care under Medicaid if they have a yearly family income for two individuals (herself and her unborn child) below $15,441.36 (in 2002 dollars).[6]

However, in some states this income cutoff may be higher. There is a second group of eligibility categories set at the federal level under Medicaid called "categorically related." This group of categories is "optional," meaning that federal funds for partial reimbursement are available for these categories but states are not required to cover those who are eligible under these categories. As of 2002, pregnant women whose family income is between 133 and 185 percent of the poverty line fall within this group.[7] Many states have opted to utilize this higher cutoff, so that, as of 2002, single pregnant women in several states are eligible for Medicaid benefits if they have an annual family income for two individuals (herself and her unborn child) below $21,478.56 (that is, 185 percent of the poverty line).[8] However, some states have also used their own funds to set this limit even higher. For instance, California, the District of Columbia, Illinois, and Vermont have set their income cutoff at 200 percent of the poverty line (a $23,220 yearly limit for a single pregnant woman), while Georgia, Rhode Island, and Minnesota have set their limits at between 235 and 275 percent of the poverty line (implying a yearly limit ranging between $27,283.44 and $31,927.56 for a single pregnant woman).[9]

While the initiatives of some states to extend benefits to larger numbers of women with these optional income standards is certainly to be commended, the larger implication of these optional federal categories is a great deal of variation across states in women's access to prenatal care. That is, there are significant gaps in Medicaid coverage since a woman living near the poverty line in one state may be eligible for prenatal care under Medicaid, while a woman with the same income living in a neighboring state may be denied.[10] While we certainly support the existing policy of extending Medicaid benefits to higher-income women by counting single pregnant women as "two," these gaps resulting from state variations are troubling. We would like to see this "optional" category of pregnant women living between 133 and 185 percent of the poverty line treated as a "mandatory" category so that all states would be required to extend benefits to this group. According to our findings, women in this income category, while technically not "poor," are still subject to a relatively high risk of giving birth to a low-birth-weight baby.

Finally, there is a third Medicaid eligibility group at the federal level, the "medically needy." This optional eligibility group allows states to extend Medicaid eligibility to people who would be eligible under either the mandatory or optional groups except that their income and resources are above the eligibility level set by their state. People can qualify under this option if they can show that, after subtracting medical expenses from their income, their resources are at or below the state's income cutoff. As of 2000, however, only 38 states had elected to have a "medically needy" program.[11]

We believe that this "medically needy" category could be used to integrate family medical histories into existing Medicaid eligibility frameworks. Higher-income parents with a family history of low birth weight (that is, a low-birth-weight birth either on the mother's or the father's side or a prior low-birth-weight birth to either parent) may be able to increase their health care resources and thus reduce their chances of a low-birth-weight birth if allowed to qualify for Medicaid coverage through a system related to the "medically needy" option. Since these families are at a disproportionate risk for poor birth outcomes, there are grounds for them to be considered "medically needy," and they ought to be able to qualify for Medicaid even at higher income levels. A complication arises, however. Since we are trying to prevent poor birth outcomes, rather than dealing with them after the fact, at-risk women will not yet have encountered complications. That is, they will not have the excessive medical costs that are required to be eligible for the "medically needy" option. Thus, here we must calculate, perhaps, the average cost of low-birth-weight complications within a specified time period, and women with incomes that are higher than the state cutoff by approximately this amount could be eligible for Medicaid.

Supplemental Nutrition Program for Women, Infants, and Children (WIC). Diet and access to nutritious food vary substantially across income categories, and federal and state programs have been devised to help poor pregnant women gain greater access to good food. One of the most notable among these programs is the Supplemental Nutrition Program for Women, Infants, and Children (WIC), a federal program that seeks to improve infant health through intervention in the prenatal period. Focusing on nutrition, WIC distributes food, food vouchers, or food checks to eligible pregnant, breast-feeding, and postpartum women, infants, and children up to the age of five, providing specific nutrients known to be missing in the diets of each of these populations.

WIC, primarily through its eligibility criteria, comes closer than almost any other state or federal welfare program (except for maybe Supplemental Security Income, which we will discuss later) to paying systematic attention to both biological and social risk. Eligibility for WIC benefits depends on three factors. First, participants must be pregnant or postpartum to be eligible. Second, women must also have family incomes below a minimum level. This income level is set by state agencies, but federal law requires that limits be between 100 and 185 percent of the poverty line. This means that, in fiscal year 2002, single pregnant women with yearly income below $15,892 may be eligible for WIC benefits.[12] There is no attention to pregnancies in the determination of "need" in these income criteria, so pregnant women count as one individual, rather than two as is the case with Medicaid. However, many higher-income pregnant women are still eligible for WIC benefits because all persons who participate in certain other benefit programs—such as Medicaid[13]—automatically meet the income eligibility criteria of WIC.[14] Thus, single pregnant women who are eligible for Medicaid under its policy of taking pregnancies into account will also be eligible for WIC. While fetuses are not explicitly taken into account in WIC eligibility, they can be indirectly accounted for via Medicaid eligibility.

Third, to be eligible for WIC benefits participants must be determined to be "at nutritional risk" based on a medical and/or nutritional assessment by a "competent professional authority," such as a physician, nutritionist, or nurse. The criteria that WIC uses to establish nutritional risk for women include abnormal weight-to-height ratios, abnormal levels in blood tests, the presence of pregnancy-induced conditions (such as toxemia or preeclampsia), and prior birth complications (such as miscarriage or stillbirth—low birth weight is not included here).[15] Thus through the design of its eligibility standards, WIC simultaneously considers social and biological categories of risk.

As we discussed in chapter 3, evidence on the effects of nutritional and prenatal intervention on birth weight and other aspects of infant health in the U.S. population is rather mixed.[16] Yet most evidence suggests that WIC is a highly effective program. Estimates based on meta-analysis suggest that WIC participation reduces rates of low birth weight by 25 percent and rates of very low birth weight by 44 percent.[17]

While unobserved differences between people who receive WIC and those who do not may be partially responsible for this difference, it still appears that WIC is doing at least something right. Based on a wide, but of course incomplete and not entirely systematic, review of the literature on this topic, it seems to us that WIC takes two approaches that are not necessarily taken in other programs. The first is education. By offering mandatory seminars on nutrition, WIC may actually work to change women's habits in positive ways, and this likely has a stronger effect on birth outcomes than food supplements alone would. The second is the biological specificity that WIC incorporates into its program. By using biological criteria to establish risk, WIC offers appropriate services to those women who need them most and are therefore the most likely to benefit. It thus appears that, drawing on existing knowledge of both social situations and biological processes, WIC is able to avoid some of the pitfalls that plague other prenatal programs.

As a federal grant program, WIC begins each fiscal year with an annual funding level set by Congress and must work within this budget. Thus the number of persons served by WIC depends on the total funds available and the allocation of funds to each agency. When a local WIC agency begins to reach the maximum participation level within available funds, a system of priorities is followed in allocating remaining resources to eligible applicants. There are seven priority categories, the highest of which is given to pregnant and breast-feeding women and infants at medically based nutritional risk (that is, nutritional risk documented by a medical condition, such as anemia). Lower priority is given to postpartum women who are not breast-feeding and current participants who, without WIC benefits, could continue to have medical and/or dietary problems. Once resources become scarce, these priority codes must be followed, and all applicants in the higher-priority category must be served before applicants in the lower-priority codes.[18]

Working within these existing eligibility and priority guidelines, it seems that family legacies of low birth weight could play an important part in WIC. In particular, a family history of low birth weight could be included as a factor in determining nutritional risk. As policy currently stands, WIC already considers a history of pregnancy complications (namely, miscarriages or stillbirths) to be indicative of nutritional risk. A history of low birth weight on either the mother's or father's side, as well as the mother having a prior low-birth-weight birth, could simply be added to this list of prior conditions indicating nutritional risk. Additionally, such histories of low birth weight could be used to qualify applicants for high-priority categories in times of scarcity. In other words, we believe that family histories of low birth weight should be included in the first WIC priority level that is instituted when funds are low.

This additional biological specificity in WIC guidelines could prove quite cost-effective. A low-birth-weight birth is extremely expensive in terms of health care. In 1988 (the most recent year for which we found data),[19] the average health care cost during the first year of life for a normal-birth-weight baby was $1,900. For a low-birth-weight infant born in the same year, the average cost of health care was $15,000. Meanwhile, for an extremely-low-birth-weight infant the average cost of health care totaled $32,000.[20] Since 1988 the costs associated with low birth weight have likely only risen as technology has improved and become more expensive. Comparing the cost of preventive services—in this case, prenatal WIC benefits—to the cost of treating diseases associated with low birth weight that began in the first 60 days of life with Medicaid, researchers have found that for every dollar spent on prevention, the associated governmental savings in Medicaid costs ranged from $2.98 to $4.75, depending on the state.[21] Thus, after-the-fact efforts to reduce the suffering associated with low birth weight cost three to four times WIC's preventive efforts. Working to improve birth outcomes clearly saves money down the road, and further targeting resources to those families at the greatest biological risk will likely only increase the efficiency and savings associated with preventive efforts.

At the same time, it is unclear whether these benefits of prenatal nutrition programs—or prenatal programs more generally—will be consistent across different causes of low birth weight. There is reason to believe, for instance, that cases of low birth weight caused by intrauterine growth retardation (IUGR) may be more sensitive to preventive efforts than cases of low birth weight resulting from preterm delivery. Jeffrey Kallan has found that race differences in the risk of low birth weight can be accounted for more effectively by differences in rates of IUGR than by differences in rates of preterm delivery. According to this analysis, the difference occurs primarily because IUGR appears to be more sensitive to immediate sociodemographic and behavioral factors (e.g., marital status—which is likely a reflection of socioeconomic status—and smoking behavior) than preterm delivery (which appears more sensitive to prepregnancy health conditions, such as hypertension or pelvic inflammatory disease).[22] Thus, it seems that prenatal preventive programs that precisely address socioeconomic status and behavior during pregnancy would be more effective at reducing IUGR than at reducing preterm deliveries.

Temporary Assistance for Needy Families. Beyond direct services, poor pregnant women also need money. Health care and nutritional services are important, but having a decent income is also crucial. A disposable income allows one to secure adequate housing and buy clothing as well as other necessities. An adequate income also provides coverage in the case of unexpected events like an illness, divorce, or loss of a job. It also reduces stress that may affect perinatal outcomes. Thus, beyond the direct services offered under Medicaid and WIC, government cash assistance programs can also be critical in preventing low birth weight among poor women.

Temporary Assistance for Needy Families (TANF), the central government cash assistance program, can be one of the main ways that the poor supplement or obtain income. As such, it could potentially play a very important role in targeting economic resources toward pregnant women. However, the status of pregnant women and fetuses within TANF is rather ambiguous. The main categorical criterion under TANF requires that one be part of a family with children in order to receive benefits. Pregnancies in many cases are assumed to meet this criterion. As of 1999, 32 states treat pregnant women who are not already caring for children as eligible for TANF. But in the majority of cases (22 of the 32 states) this eligibility applies only to the last trimester of a pregnancy (in several of these 22 states such eligibility applies only to the very last month of a pregnancy).[23] Under these guidelines (particularly when eligibility applies only to the last month of a pregnancy), it would seem that administrators are more concerned with ensuring that benefits are in place for the child after birth, rather than for his or her prenatal development. It is, indeed, doubtful that receiving TANF benefits only in the last trimester of pregnancy can have any real effect on the health of fetuses or on birth outcomes.

Beyond the central categorical criterion limiting benefits to families with children, families must also have incomes (and in most states assets) below a given level. Precisely how income eligibility is determined varies significantly across states. Suffice it to say that in the vast majority of states families must pass needs-based income tests. That is, families must have a "countable income" (income after deductions) that falls below the states' net income limits for a family of that size.[24] While most states do not use the federal poverty line to determine income eligibility for TANF, the needs-based income tests used for TANF are similar to the federal poverty line in that they determine need based on what is assumed to be the cost of living for a family of a given size. Based on data from 2002, no states consider pregnancies in determining these income eligibility limits.[25] That is, there are no instances in TANF policy in which pregnant women are counted as "two" in determining a family's size and, hence, level of need.

Further, under TANF, once income eligibility criteria are passed, benefit levels also depend on family size. In the majority of cases (35 states), a family's benefits amount is the difference between its "countable income" and the state's maximum benefit level for a family of its size.[26] Again, however, pregnancies are given no special consideration in determining maximum benefit levels. That is, since family size is not assumed to vary with pregnancy status, maximum benefit levels do not take pregnancies into account.

TANF stands in a very good position to target economic resources toward pregnant women. Since it is one of the central cash assistance programs for poor families and since eligibility and benefits vary by family size, accounting for pregnancies would require relatively little change in policy procedures and could have far-reaching implications. Yet at this point, TANF seems to make little effort in this direction. Pregnancies are given almost no attention if children are already present, and if children are not already present, benefits become available so late in a pregnancy that they can have little effect. We would like to see this situation changed in two ways. First, we would like to see pregnant women without any children become eligible for TANF during the first month of their pregnancy in all states. And second, we would like to see pregnant women counted as two individuals in the assessment of family size under TANF so that income eligibility levels and maximum benefit levels will be raised for pregnant women.

There are two factors, however, that may complicate implementation of these suggestions. Since TANF is a program targeted at families with children, the term *children* is explicit in this program. This could make our suggestion to count pregnancies in assessments of family size rather controversial, potentially leading to debates over abortion comparable to those that emerged with Bush's SCHIP proposal. As we mentioned above, however, we must balance the potential good that can result from targeting resources at pregnant women against such potential problems, and we cannot let possible misinterpretations block efforts to prevent low birth weight.

In addition, those who are particularly concerned over "perverse incentives" provided by cash benefits may argue that counting pregnancies in the determination of eligibility and benefits would encourage "undesirable" behaviors—particularly nonmarital fertility—among women receiving TANF. There has indeed been concern among politicians, policymakers, and the public (particularly under the former cash assistance program, Aid to Families with Dependent Children) that incremental increases in cash assistance corresponding to family size lead women—often while unmarried—to have additional children. Some states have responded to these concerns by implementing "family caps" that "freeze" benefit levels at a given family size so that children conceived or born while the family is receiving cash assistance are not eligible for TANF.[27] In this case, for the purposes of TANF, family size is not considered to increase with this child. Our suggestion to make benefits more generous for pregnant women could be interpreted by some as a "perverse incentive" encouraging single women to conceive children. Because of such concern, states that already have "family cap" policies in place would seem relatively unlikely to adopt our suggestion of increasing benefits in cases of pregnancy.

In addressing this potential criticism of our suggestions, we stress that there is no decisive evidence supporting these claims that cash benefits encourage women to have children while unmarried. Despite the great deal of publicity these claims have received, empirical evidence clearly showing that decisions about fertility are sensitive to cash assistance policies is sparse.[28] Further, policies such as family caps that seek to discourage women from having children essentially punish children for their parents' behavior. Policies such as these increase the chances that children will live in poverty—both prenatally and during childhood—and thus, according to our results, likely jeopardize children's long-term outcomes. This implies that policies that work to reduce pregnant women and children's economic resources will likely have long-term negative consequences that may prove more costly in the long run, as familial cycles of poverty and poor health are maintained, than the more immediate expenditures associated with TANF.[29]

The Earned Income Tax Credit and the Child Tax Credit. While often not considered part of social welfare policy, tax credits are another important way to target resources at pregnant women. Here we are concerned primarily with credits that are already designed to vary depending on the number of children in a family. The first of these is the Earned Income Tax Credit (EITC), which targets low-wage earners (in 2001 this meant a modified adjusted gross annual income less than $27,413 for a taxpayer with one child and a modified adjusted gross annual income less than $31,152 for a taxpayer with more than one child).[30] Tax credits are generally an amount individuals can subtract from the taxes they owe for such expenses as child care or care for an elderly or disabled person. The EITC, however, is a special class of tax credit—a refundable credit—that allows people who have an income below the taxation threshold to receive the credit as a direct payment from the U.S. Treasury. If, however, the person has an income above the taxation threshold, the credit is simply subtracted from what he or she owes, as with most other tax credits.

According to 2001 tax law, some eligible employees with at least one child living with them may be entitled to receive advance EITC payments in their paychecks.[31] In this case, the employer simply pays part of the credit to the employee in advance throughout the year, and the taxpayer claims the rest when filing his or her federal tax return. In this way, the EITC can be another way that poor or near-poor women may increase their earnings. If pregnant women are allowed to include their pregnancy as a "child" in the calculations of their advanced tax credits, they can likely increase in their earnings while pregnant.

The Child Tax Credit has slightly different criteria but is still another way that pregnant women may increase their disposable income. In order to be eligible for the Child Tax Credit, one must have a dependent child who is a U.S. citizen and must have a modified adjusted gross yearly income below a certain amount (in 2001, the credit began to phase out at $110,000 for married couples filing jointly and at $75,000 for single heads of household).[32] Provided one has met these criteria, one can then reduce one's tax liability by $500 for every qualifying child (as of 2001).[33] For individuals who have one or two qualifying children, the Child Tax Credit (unlike the EITC) is nonrefundable, which means that people cannot claim any credit beyond their liability. However, if individuals have three or more qualifying children and are not able to claim the full Child Tax Credit because of low earnings, they can claim the Additional Child Tax Credit, which is refundable. In this case, low-wage taxpayers with at least three kids can receive a direct cash transfer from the U.S. Treasury, as with the EITC.

As of 2001, employees cannot claim an advance on the Child Tax Credit or the Additional Child Tax Credit, so it is not—yet, at least—possible for employees to have their employers reduce withholding to reflect the credit.[34] Provided that this policy can be changed, though, the Child Tax Credit may also be used to target resources at pregnant women. As with the EITC, if the child tax credit is extended to pregnant women so that they may count their pregnancy as a "child" in the calculation of their taxes, we may increase the disposable income of pregnant women, thereby reducing the likelihood of low birth weight.

Tax fraud is a complication that may accompany these advanced tax credits. It is surely harder to verify the existence of a pregnancy than it is to verify the existence of a child. Therefore, some individuals may be tempted to falsely state they are pregnant in order claim the credit and reduce their withholdings. It seems that the simplest way to avoid this is to make people liable for the credit if there is not a birth (a stillbirth or live birth) or a medically certified miscarriage[35] within approximately nine months following the request for advanced credit.

In sum, we have suggested that—in cases in which existing policy supports biological specificity (here we considered the cases of Medicaid and WIC)—a family history of low birth weight should qualify pregnant women for special statuses in social programs. We have further suggested that—in cases in which programs have less room for such particularities (as with TANF and tax credits)—all pregnancies should be considered qualifying events that increase a family's size in cost-of-living calculations. Thus, in some cases our suggestions have been biologically specific, while in others they have been more universal. This dual tendency, rather than being an inconsistency, may be a strength of our suggestions since it will likely be easier to draw sustained public support for these expansions if they have elements that offer resources to and appeal to larger groups in society (beyond those facing particular biological risk factors like low birth weight). Further, joining our biologically specific suggestions with more general suggestions, we may reduce some of the emphasis placed on heritability in these discussions and, thus, possibly avoid some of the controversies or misinterpretations around genetics that we discussed above.

Before concluding this discussion of prevention, we should at least begin to address the question of how much we can expect from these proposals—or from prenatal programs in general. As our analyses have shown, extra dollars during pregnancies can help prevent poor birth outcomes (when a biological risk is present). But it would seem naïve to expect that raising poor pregnant women's resources and thus reducing inequalities for nine-month periods would counteract lifetimes and generations of starker inequalities. However, as mentioned above in our discussion of IUGR and preterm deliveries, some conditions may be more sensitive to immediate social situations, and thus more sensitive to preventive efforts, than other conditions that result from longer-term inequalities.

INTERVENTION

Having examined the question of how we might more effectively prevent low birth weight,.it is now time to consider how we might reduce the negative consequences of low birth weight in cases when it cannot be avoided. Our results have shown that low birth weight has both short-term and long-term effects. For those low-birth-weight babies who avoid the immediate risk of infant mortality that we documented in our twin analysis, having been born low birth weight can significantly hinder educational attainment—increasing the chances of grade retention, enrollment in special education, and diagnosis as learning disabled and decreasing the chances of timely high school graduation. Further, we have some evidence to suggest that these very-long-term consequences may be sensitive to socioeconomic status. Although, as we discussed before, these results are not immune from selection bias, our models did show that, when household incomes reach five times the poverty level, the negative effects of low birth weight are reduced.

These longer- and shorter-term consequences of low birth weight have two implications that we must consider. First, there is the general question of what resources are available to low-birth-weight children for intervening in any interactive effects of poverty and low birth weight. Because of their high risk for disability and poverty, low-birth-weight children are a population that will frequently need to rely on federal assistance programs. In the following discussion we will, therefore, briefly review and make some suggestions regarding the cash assistance programs most applicable to low-birth-weight children. That is, we will consider what particular aspects of these programs may be altered to better target resources toward children born low birth weight.

Second, there is the more specific matter of low birth weight and education. Our finding that low birth weight has long-term educational consequences implies that it ought to be considered a risk factor throughout childhood and into young adulthood. Most programs for at-risk children currently pay considerable attention to biological and social risk factors at early ages. However, as children age, these programs tend to focus less on the etiologies of children's problems than on the problems themselves. For instance, while preschool programs such as the Infant Health and Development Program (IHDP) or Head Start pay considerable attention to the social and biological factors that place children at risk, special education programs in elementary school and high school are far less concerned with the factors leading to disabilities and than with managing the disabilities themselves. We believe there is an important place for understanding and addressing risk factors, such as low birth weight, over the entire course of a child's education.

In some respects, this suggestion that low birth weight be considered a risk factor through childhood and young adulthood requires that we reconsider how we understand child development. A large part of the reason that we witness this shift in attention from risk factors at early ages to disabilities at later ages is that many developmental theories have highlighted critical periods of rapid growth and change in young ages at the expense of attention to growth and change at older ages.[36] Thus it has often been assumed that risk factors matter more at young ages than at older ages. That is, because developmental theory has emphasized critical periods of development in young ages, it has often been assumed (both implicitly and explicitly) that biological and environmental risk will be more damaging at earlier ages. In some cases, it is even assumed that the "damage has been done" by the time a child reaches a certain age. This approach can often be found in low-birth-weight analysis, as researchers have often assumed that the importance of low birth weight dwindles with age. Analyses of low birth weight have often been limited to early ages, repeatedly drawing comparisons between low-birth-weight and normal-birth-weight infants and toddlers, and rarely drawing such comparisons in school-age children or teenagers.[37]

In the following discussion, we offer the contrary argument that child development is a long-term and multifaceted process that cannot be contained within the early years or attributed exclusively to biological or social conditions. As the long-term process of maturing unfolds over the years of childhood and young adulthood, there are repeated and varied interactions between biological dispositions and environment. At younger ages, for instance, prematurity and environmental hazards, like an inadequate diet or poor neighborhood, may interact with one another, leading to failure to thrive. At older ages, learning disabilities related to birth weight may combine with bad labor market conditions to make low-birth-weight teenagers more likely to drop out of high school than normal-birth-weight teenagers. Rather than a "cumulative" framework for child development, we suggest an "interlocking" one, in which early conditions (such as birth weight) do not get subsumed within later risk factors or permanently and decisively change children's developmental trajectories. Rather, later childhood conditions may affect how earlier ones express themselves (or not). Early childhood conditions, likewise, may appear to diminish in importance over time, but then may reassert themselves later on, if other biological conditions or social stressors are manifested.

The problem, however, in assuming such a complicated biosocial model of child development is that the specific role of particular risk factors—such as low birth weight—can be ambiguous. As the biological factors associated with low birth weight interact in varied ways with multiple environmental factors, we would expect to find—indeed, do find—a large diversity in the types and severities of disabilities faced by children born low birth weight. Thus, what can low birth weight really contribute as a risk factor, particularly at older ages when diversity should be greatest? In some respects, this is a difficult question to answer. Low birth weight is associated with mild behavioral problems but also with blindness and cerebral palsy. Certainly not all of these very different conditions can be lumped together. Yet low birth weight is a common factor across many disabilities and as such may matter in the treatment of these disabilities.

As we will argue in greater detail below, we believe that awareness of low-birth-weight status may help in the identification and treatment of disabilities. For instance, knowing that a child was born low birth weight and therefore (as chapter 4 shows) is at an increased risk for a learning impairment may help teachers, physicians, and parents be on the lookout for potential developmental problems. Given our evidence documenting the long-term consequences of low birth weight, there is also reason to suspect that responses to treatments for various disabilities may vary by birth weight. For example, a low-birth-weight child who has attention deficit hyperactivity disorder or who suffers from some of the problems associated with autism may respond differently to treatments than a child with these conditions who is not low birth weight. We cannot say with any definitiveness, of course, that this is the case, but our evidence of the long-term educational consequences of low birth weight does suggest that low birth weight may have a further role to play in refining treatments. Researchers, physicians, therapists, and others should keep low birth weight in mind as a factor when assessing the effectiveness and appropriateness of treatment for disabilities.

Before proceeding, it is also important to note that the approach we take to risk factors and child development in this discussion may be expanded to apply beyond the particular case of low birth weight. Other disabilities and developmental problems whose sequelae we would expect to be sensitive to environmental factors—mental retardation may be an example—may also benefit from longer-term attention paid to social and biological etiologies. By continuing to keep the early causes of various disabilities—whether prematurity, lead poisoning, or even malnutrition—in mind as children age, we may be able to better target and refine the treatments that we currently have for disabilities.

Disposable Income and Cash Assistance

As has been noted several times in this book, money matters. Adequate economic resources are crucial for creating a positive environment for children. A reasonable income allows parents to secure good housing in a safe neighborhood, obtain nutritious food and educational toys, and not least important, reduce the stress on themselves, facilitating positive and warm interactions with their children.[38] Thus, federal cash assistance—namely, TANF and Supplemental Security Income (SSI)—remains one of the central ways that we may curb the effects of low birth weight and economic impoverishment on children.

As the main federal cash assistance program for children, TANF will likely play an important role in the well-being of low-birth-weight children. Aspects of the TANF program, however, while potentially troubling for all children, may be particularly problematic for low-birth-weight children. These aspects generally stem from the work requirements faced by parents who receive TANF benefits. Under TANF legislation, 50 percent of all families receiving benefits in the state must work or participate in work-related activities (which range from vocational education to community service, depending on the state in question). According to these provisions, single parents are required to work 30 hours per week, while two-parent families are required to work 35 to 55 hours per week.[39]

States enjoy a fair amount of discretion in how to impose these general federal requirements. That is, states generally make the call as to when and why a family may be excused from the work requirements. While many states (34 as of 2000) exempt individuals with disabilities or temporary illness or incapacity from TANF work requirements, fewer states (only 28 as of 2000) allow such exemptions if another individual in the household is disabled.[40] This tendency is troubling for our population of low-birth-weight children since there is a higher-than-average chance that parents in this population will be caring for a disabled child and, therefore, may not be able to comply with TANF work requirements. That is, even if a parent is in excellent health, the illnesses or disabilities found in low-birth-weight children can present a sizable barrier to employment that may not be addressed in a given state's TANF exemption policies. This situation may place low-birth-weight children at a particularly high risk of losing their TANF benefits because of sanctions.

Although we do not have data on how many children receiving TANF benefits were born low birth weight, we do know that a high percentage of WIC recipients (between 11.6 and 13.1 percent, depending on the data set used) were born low birth weight. Since many families receiving WIC benefits also receive TANF assistance (up to 70.1 percent, again depending on the data set), we would expect to see a considerable portion of TANF families with low-birth-weight children.[41] Thus, here we see low-birth-weight children in a particularly vulnerable position with respect to TANF. Children born low birth weight—precisely those children in the greatest need of economic resources and a positive environment—are at disproportionately high risk of being denied benefits because of conditions related to their birth weight. To address this situation, we would like to see all states allow exemptions from work requirements if a child's disability presents a significant barrier to employment.

Further questions surrounding TANF work requirements relate to the quality and availability of child care. Requirements that parents work create an obvious need for someone to look after children living in TANF families. The government has not entirely failed to recognize this need and with the enactment of TANF in 1996 there was a $600 million (or 27 percent) increase over prior federal spending on child care for low-income families.[42] Despite this increase, though, we still do not find the demand for child care satisfied. A study of child care in 13 states that encompass half the U.S. population found that, even with states drawing down the maximum level of funds from the federal government, assistance could be provided to at most about half of the low-income children with parents seeking child care assistance. While this is a substantial improvement over the one-third of children who would have been covered in the pre-TANF programs, we are still far from universal coverage.[43]

Beyond the question of how many children can be served is the problem of the quality of care. Covering as many families as possible may seem ideal, but working within finite budgets, such a far reach would also lead to lower reimbursement rates for individual families and would limit parents' choices of providers, likely lowering the quality of care. While lower reimbursement rates allow states to stretch the available funds over a greater number of children, they also may make it more difficult for families to find good providers who will accept the lower rate.[44] While these dilemmas surrounding child care are clearly a problem for all children, they may pose particular risk for low-birth-weight children. Since these children, already facing biological risk, may be particularly sensitive to any harmful aspects of their environments, inadequate—or even less than ideal—child care may heighten any negative effects of low birth weight. Thus again we find low-birth-weight children in an especially vulnerable position with regard to TANF's work requirements.

Another federal cash assistance program that is highly relevant to the economic conditions of low-birth-weight children is SSI. Under this program, disabled children younger than 18 who come from homes with limited incomes and resources are eligible for up to $545 per month (as of 2002) in cash assistance.[45] Since 2000, disability in children has been defined as "a medically determinable physical or mental impairment or combination of impairments that cause marked or severe functional limitation, and that can be expected to last for a continuous period of not less than 12 months."[46] This definition is somewhat stricter than the one in effect prior to the 1996 welfare reform, since it does not consider developmental lags to be a disability. With the 1996 reform, the Individual Functional Assessment Test, which was used to document developmental deficiencies, was eliminated, leaving only those children with more severe disabilities who could qualify through a master medical list eligible for SSI.[47]

Overall, it has been estimated that this change in the definition of disability reduced the 1996 SSI caseload by approximately 15 percent.[48] While we do not have data available on the number of SSI children who were born low birth weight, this change has probably meant that now it is only extremely-low-birth-weight children with more severe complications who can qualify for SSI. Slightly larger low-birth-weight children who do not suffer from severe disabilities (such as cerebral palsy or blindness) but are still likely to have significant developmental deficiencies would seem, in contrast, to be the most likely to have lost benefits with the 1996 reform. Since SSI benefits can be sizable for low-income families, such loss of eligibility has likely led to a significant decline in the standard of living among these families. It has been estimated, for instance, that losing SSI benefits because of the 1996 reform may have eliminated approximately 30 percent of a poor family's income.[49] Given the role that income can play in counteracting the biological deficiencies associated with low birth weight, such a loss likely poses a significant threat to low-birth-weight children, making them more vulnerable to the biological risk factors they face. Since we find some evidence to suggest that higher incomes in childhood have long-term educational payoffs, it would seem that reinvesting funds so that low-birth-weight children with developmental lags can be covered with SSI would be a wise and efficient use of federal money.[50]

The Education of Low-Birth-Weight Children

Beyond the question of individual household incomes, we must also consider how the formal education system may be used to maximize the potential of low-birth-weight children. As we mentioned before, in contrast to our results documenting the long-term educational disadvantage faced by low-birth-weight children, most educational programs that take birth weight into account and provide the most comprehensive intervention services are limited to very young ages. Indeed, a distinct split can be found between early education and later education in terms of the way birth weight and environmental factors figure into the discussion. At young ages, birth weight and environmental disadvantage are given important etiological roles and are explicitly considered in the assessment and treatment of impairments, such as developmental lags or illnesses. At older ages, however, when these same impairments are renamed as learning or physical disabilities, impairments become self-contained and etiology is moved to the periphery. In the following discussion, after reviewing the strengths and weaknesses of early education programs, we consider whether this tendency is problematic. That is, could attention to the birth weight status of older children contribute to the design of their education?

The Early Years: Low Birth Weight–Specific Intervention and Head Start. The most notable birth weight–specific intervention programs have proceeded in a relatively logical fashion, each one building on the experiences (and shortcomings) of the previous program. The first program, called the Abecedarian Project, was begun in the mid-1980s and offered intensive, high-quality preschool programs (along with medical and nutritional support) beginning shortly after birth and continuing until the child entered kindergarten. The direct successor to the Abecedarian Project, called Project CARE, was designed to test whether home-based intervention that taught mothers how to provide good developmental stimulation for their infants and toddlers might be more effective than center-based intervention.[51] The third program, the Infant Health and Development Program (IHDP), was much larger than the first two and culminated in a great deal of research. This program essentially combined the center-based and family-based approaches of the two previous programs by offering low-birth-weight infants and their families pediatric follow-ups, family support through home visits and parent support groups, and intensive, high-quality preschool services.[52]

These major birth weight–specific programs seem quite comprehensive, but are they effective? In terms of IQ scores and behavioral problems, these interventions appear quite helpful. Health, however, is another story. Considering evidence from the IHDP, since it is the most comprehensive program and was the most thoroughly researched, we see that mean IQ scores were significantly higher for the infants who received the full intervention as compared to the infants who were in the control group. Behavioral problems were also far less prevalent among the infants who participated in the intervention. The odds of a child scoring in the range that would imply clinically evident behavioral problems in the control group was approximately twice that in the intervention group. Health outcomes for infants in the intervention group, however, were not so positive. Comparing children with similar birth weights, participating in the intervention program was associated with higher morbidity scores.[53] Researchers have argued, however, that this outcome may be the result of reporting bias or the more intensive health surveillance of the intervention infants.[54]

While this evidence clearly suggests that, overall, intervention has a positive effect on the early development of low-birth-weight infants, other evidence suggests that intervention does not lead to universally positive returns. Researchers following infants who participated in the IHDP have found that, while the intervention services were generally quite helpful, they were most effective for larger low-birth-weight children coming from more disadvantaged homes. Both black and white children whose mothers had at most a high school degree exhibited greater cognitive benefits from intervention than children whose mothers had attended college.[55] In the cases of low maternal education, the home environment is likely less enriched to begin with, and therefore, the services offered by the program probably made a larger difference to these children. Birth weight also affected response to treatment, so that children born with higher weights benefited more from intervention services than children born smaller.[56] Here we are likely witnessing a biosocial interaction, such that, once biological deficits become severe enough, environmental influences become less important. Jeanne Brooks-Gunn and her colleagues have even suggested that these mediating factors of maternal education and birth weight may be translated into policy so that, in times of fiscal constraint, intervention may be targeted at children who stand to benefit the most.[57]

In addition to these intervention programs that specifically target low-birth-weight children, there are more general programs for disabled children that can be quite important for our low-birth-weight population. Operating under the Individuals with Disabilities Education Act (IDEA) are two federal programs that serve disabled preschool children. For very young children there is the Infants and Toddlers with Disabilities Program (often referred to simply as "early intervention"), through which the federal government provides grants to states for services for disabled children aged birth through two. Under this program, states must provide services (ranging from physical and speech therapy to assistive technology services and family training) to all age-appropriate children who are experiencing a developmental delay or who have a diagnosed physical or mental condition that is likely to lead to a developmental delay.[58] The legislation guiding this program strongly emphasizes the prevention of further disability. For instance, according to Congress, the goals of this program include minimizing the need for later special education and institutionalization.[59]

Prior to the establishment of this federal early intervention program in 1986, a variety of public and private agencies were providing services to preschool children with disabilities. When designing the Infants and Toddlers with Disabilities Program, Congress sought to build on this existing informal structure.[60] Therefore, the federal government allows for significant variation in the specifics of these programs across states—perhaps most starkly with regard to eligibility criteria. As mentioned above, federal legislation requires that states serve all infants and toddlers with a developmental delay or a physical and mental condition that will likely result in a developmental delay.[61] However, the legislation allows states to decide whether they will serve children who are at risk for but do not yet exhibit such a substantial developmental delay.[62] Thus, there is considerable variation across states in how far these programs will reach. Low-birth-weight children are likely to be particularly affected by this state variation since low birth weight, according to Congress, is one of the main biological factors that may be used to tag a child as at risk.[63] This means that, while some states may specifically include children born low birth weight in this program by having services for at-risk children in general, other states may not. In cases when states do not serve at-risk children, the presence of other handicaps that frequently accompany low birth weight (such as cerebral palsy or blindness) would likely be necessary for children to qualify for this program.

A second program operating under IDEA that serves young children with disabilities is the Preschool Grants Program. Through this program the federal government provides grants to states to make special education and related services available to disabled children ages three though five. While the general legislative structure of this program is similar to that of the Infants and Toddlers with Disabilities Program, this Preschool Grants Program takes a different approach to eligibility and services that appears to reflect different philosophies surrounding the age groups served by these programs. As we discussed above, we often find a diminished emphasis placed on prevention and development in programs that serve older children, and this tendency is particularly clear if we compare these two federal programs.

While the Infants and Toddlers with Disabilities Program defines disability with special attention to developmental delays (in the hope of preventing further delay), the Preschool Grants Program uses, instead, disability criteria similar to those used in special education assessment for older children.[64] Further, while the Infants and Toddlers with Disabilities Program allowed for state discretion in serving at-risk children, with attention to particular risk factors (like low birth weight), the Preschool Grants Program allows similar state discretion in serving children with developmental delays.[65] Thus, it seems that there is a shift in the concerns that guide these two programs. While the Infants and Toddlers with Disabilities Program gave developmental delays primary importance and secondary priority to risk factors, the Preschool Grants Program gives disabilities themselves primary importance, developmental delays secondary priority, and risk factors no explicit attention at all.

Beyond this variation in eligibility criteria, the two programs also vary in the settings in which services are offered. While most services under the Infants and Toddlers with Disabilities Program are rendered in the home, most Preschool Grants Program services take place in a preschool setting. Almost 80 percent of the youngsters with disabilities served under this program are placed in a preschool classroom (either a general education or special education class).[66] While this shift is likely quite appropriate given the age difference between the two groups of children served, there is further the question of parents' roles in these programs. It is far more likely that parents will learn more about managing their children's disabilities when participating in the Infants and Toddlers with Disabilities Program than in the Preschool Grants Program.

How effective and appropriate are these more general early intervention programs for low-birth-weight children? Unfortunately, this is not an easy question to answer—mainly because the necessary data do not yet exist. Although these programs were established in 1986, we do not witness a significant rise in the number of children participating in them until around 1997.[67] This has meant that it was only recently that Congress began allocating significant funds for research on these programs. As of 2002, the two national surveys tracking these programs remain in preliminary stages. The National Early Intervention Longitudinal Study (NEILS), which tracks children participating in the Infants and Toddlers with Disabilities Program, has only made available preliminary descriptive data on the population served by this program. The Pre-Elementary Education Longitudinal Study, which will track three-to-five-year-old children receiving special education services, has not yet begun collecting data due to budgetary constraints. Thus it is currently unclear how these programs relate to our concerns with the long-term educational outcomes of low-birth-weight children.

At this point we can note only that low birth weight appears to play an important role in the Infants and Toddlers with Disabilities Program. Approximately 11 percent of the children participating in the program entered specifically because of the risk posed by low birth weight. More than 11 percent of the participants were probably born low birth weight, though, since many of the alternative reasons that young children enter the program (such as prenatal exposure to drugs and alcohol or intellectual/cognitive impairment) are associated with low birth weight.[68] Further, according to preliminary data from NEILS, those children who enter the program specifically because of birth weight are more likely to do so at earlier ages and therefore may also benefit more than children entering for other reasons (like motor

impairment or speech/communication impairment), who are more likely
to enter at later ages.[69] Thus, while low birth weight is given lower status than some of the other eligibility criteria that guide the Infants and
Toddlers with Disabilities Program (because of its role as a risk factor
rather than a disability), it appears that low-birth-weight children are
still served by this program in significant numbers and may even benefit disproportionately from these services because of the early ages at
which they are likely to begin treatment.

Another early intervention program that does not specifically target
disability at all but is still quite relevant to our discussion is Head Start.
Head Start is a federally funded preschool program for economically
disadvantaged children that extends social services (such as job assistance or health care referrals) to parents as well.[70] To speak of Head
Start as a single program may be slightly misleading, though, since it
can vary significantly by location. While Head Start is administered and
at least partially funded by the federal government, it is actually run
by local public agencies, nonprofits, and school systems. All Head Start
programs are required to provide developmentally appropriate educational experiences, health screenings and referrals, nutrition education
and hot meals, and parental involvement. However, beyond these general guidelines, programs are encouraged to adapt to local needs.[71]

Considering Head Start in conjunction with birth weight–specific
programs such as IHDP and more general early special education programs such as the Infants and Toddlers with Disabilities Program, it is
useful to note parenthetically how closely linked services for low birth
weight and poverty really are. Indeed, early low-birth-weight-specific
programs were modeled after programs that targeted poor children,
such as Head Start.[72] Further, children living in poverty (as defined
by receipt of public assistance) are significantly overrepresented in the
Infants and Toddlers with Disabilities Programs.[73] While we may distinguish between biological and social factors when discussing services,
they often go hand-in-hand when services are actually implemented.

Evidence of the effectiveness of Head Start is somewhat mixed. While
Head Start appears to provide immediate and substantial gains in terms
of IQ scores and cognitive ability, most studies show that these gains
are quickly lost once children leave the program.[74] Many supporters of
Head Start have responded to these results by arguing that the program
is not only about IQ and that, in fact, its original goal was not to
improve IQs but rather to improve the overall social competence of
children. Evidence does indeed suggest the lasting effects of Head Start

are found in other areas besides IQ. For instance, studies have found that participants in Head Start were less likely to be assigned to a special education class and were somewhat less likely to be held back a grade in school.[75]

These mixed results surrounding Head Start raise the important question of how long we can expect the results associated with any of these early intervention programs to last. As noted before, child development proceeds long past the age of kindergarten, so intervention programs limited to this early time period cannot be realistically expected to have long-lasting effects. Despite this evidence, politicians who propose and support educational legislation seem to find great appeal in the quick fixes that become possible when theory limits development to short, critical periods of time. For instance, Governor Neil Goldschmidt of Oregon clearly exaggerated Head Start's possibilities when he commented that the 1990 expansion of Head Start would be the "most significant—and most effective—anti-drug, anti-crime, pro-education strategy" in America.[76] Our evidence documenting the long-term consequences of low birth weight, however, suggests that quick fixes will not provide such long-term benefits and additional educational programs will be necessary to reduce later discrepancies.

Elementary and Secondary Schools.   Once children are older and enter elementary and then secondary schools, the causal factors of birth weight and environment become even more peripheral, and the resulting disabilities occupy center stage. In other words, etiology is given little attention, and any impairments that a child may have—such as a learning disability, emotional disturbance, or physical impairment—are considered in a self-contained manner through special education programs. Special education is a large and diverse field—almost any impairment that a child may have will be addressed under this title.[77] In the following discussion, we limit our focus to higher-incidence disabilities, namely, cognitive deficits, learning disabilities, behavioral problems, emotional disturbances, and generally poorer health. There are, of course, more severe, lower-incidence disabilities, such as blindness, deafness, and cerebral palsy associated with low birth weight, which are similarly deserving of attention. However, we choose not to focus on these conditions in this discussion for a few reasons. First, such lower-incidence disabilities are often the result of quite severe biological problems, and therefore, the influence of environmental intervention is usually much more limited in scope. Further, the diagnosis and interventions for each of these more severe impairments are generally more widely recognized and agreed upon than those for higher-incidence disabilities (take, for example, the controversy surrounding the diagnosis of some learning disabilities and emotional disturbances). Therefore, the following discussion of the processes behind recognition and treatment of impairments may have more to contribute to the area of higher-incidence impairments.

Under IDEA, all students with special needs are guaranteed an Individualized Education Program (IEP) developed under the guidance of a team of parents and professionals. Because designing IEPs for all disabled students can be quite complicated, the process is generally broken down into seven steps. The first step involves referring a child for special education services. Referrals can happen in a variety of ways—parents may become concerned about a child who is not walking by age two or is not talking by age three, pediatricians may become concerned about children whose development seems delayed, or teachers may become troubled by a student displaying inappropriate behavior on a regular basis.[78]

It appears to us that our knowledge of the sequelae of low birth weight may be helpful in this referral process. Catching disabilities early can greatly improve a child's prognosis for future success. The early school years often set the stage for future educational attainment, and bad experiences or grade retention before the identification of such problems as a learning disability can lead to larger problems down the road. In addition, in some cases, there are strong connections between different impairments so that addressing one—say, a language impairment—in a timely manner will reduce the chances of further disabilities—most commonly, learning disabilities and behavioral problems. However, in many instances, identifying impairment for the purposes of referral at an early age can be quite tricky. Such is particularly the case with behavioral disorders and emotional disturbances, which tend not be noticed until later ages.[79] Since we know that low-birth-weight children are at elevated risk for several disabilities (indeed, our results from the last chapter showed that low birth weight can increase the chances that a child is diagnosed as learning disabled by 148 percent), a child's birth weight status may be helpful in the early identification of impairments. By taking etiological factors into account (in this case, birth weight), teachers, parents, and physicians may be especially watchful for signs of a disability in a child and, therefore, may better detect disabilities.

Currently, birth weight and prematurity are typically ignored after age two. In considering medical and developmental measures, physicians, therapists, and social workers will generally correct for gestation only until age two, after which such prenatal conditions are largely disregarded. This transition is comparable to daylight saving time in that the "clock" is turned forward and low-birth-weight and premature children are immediately expected to be caught up. This change around age two takes place mostly because at older ages developmental deadlines are less fixed. That is, there is a wider window of "normal" time during which a child may pass developmental milestones, so that monthly adjustments for gestational age are generally less meaningful. Yet our results documenting the long-term implications of perinatal conditions—namely, low birth weight—suggest that such factors should be kept in mind long beyond age two (even if specific corrections such as those for gestational age are less meaningful).

The next step in addressing a child's special needs involves the diagnosis and assessment of a disability. In this stage, a team of professionals, often led by a school psychologist, use an array of assessment instruments and procedures to determine whether special services are necessary and, if so, which types.[80] After this process of assessment comes the third step, identification, which is essentially the official processing and classifying of a student as disabled.[81] The fourth and fifth steps are the determination of services required and the official placement of the child in services. Essentially, in these stages professionals will design and make arrangements for the child's IEP. Given the large variation in types and severity of disabilities, there is a great deal of diversity in the ways that children will be served. In the cases of more severe disability, children are removed from general education and placed in special education classrooms. In less severe cases, students may remain in their general education classroom, leaving only a few times a week for special education services that can range from a speech pathologist or a physical therapist to a specially trained teacher simply presenting material to students in alternative ways.[82] Once special education services for students have been designed, the final steps in this process (the sixth and seventh) are begun. In these steps, teachers make decisions about the detailed aspects of curriculum and assessment and begin to carry out the child's new special education.[83]

Our results documenting the long-term educational consequences of low birth weight suggest that low birth weight matters in the long run and, therefore, there may be a role for low birth weight in designing—or more likely, refining—treatments for disabilities. However, the exact boundaries of this role remain vague at this stage. Given our results, there is a clear possibility that low-birth-weight children with particular disabilities, such as learning disabilities or hyperactivity disorders, may respond differently to treatment than other children with these same disabilities who were born normal birth weight. However, we cannot definitively state that this is the case until further research is conducted on the specific mechanisms that lead to the long-term educational differences between low-birth-weight and normal-birth-weight children. Thus at this point, it seems that low birth weight should be kept in mind in these later stages of special education implementation. That said, exactly how information about birth weight status should be used is yet to be determined.

Our suggestions that low birth weight should be considered in the identification and treatment of disabilities may have some unintended consequences. First, there is the potential that such increased attention to low-birth-weight status—particularly in the stages of identifying disabilities—may lead to stigma. While we want to catch problems early to minimize their negative ramifications, we do not want to be so hyperaware as to incorrectly diagnose children or to give low-birth-weight status the quality of a negative label that has its own harmful consequences. If a low-birth-weight child is not actually learning disabled but is diagnosed and treated as such (perhaps because of overemphasis on the roles we have laid out for birth weight), she may miss out on certain learning opportunities from which she could have benefited. But even if a low-birth-weight child is not actually diagnosed and treated as learning disabled, she may suffer if low-birth-weight status is overemphasized. For instance, we can imagine that if our suggestions about low-birth-weight status in special education were taken too far, the status could become a label that causes teachers, parents, counselors, and others to lower their expectations of low-birth-weight children (either unconsciously or consciously) and thus treat them differently.

A second unintended consequence that may result from taking these suggestions about low birth weight too far is inattention to other important risk factors relating to special education, such as an impoverished environment. Such an outcome would be, to some degree, counterproductive. We have emphasized throughout this book the importance of equal attention to biological and social risk factors, and we do not want our suggestion of increasing attention to birth weight status to detract from attention to environmental risk factors. Further attention to birth weight status in special education could possibly help in reducing the discrepancy that we found in long-term educational outcomes, but if such attention is misapplied (as is the case in either the stigmatizing outcome or inattention to other factors) the opposite effect could occur.[84]

CONCLUSION

The intergenerational cycles of low birth weight and low income that we have uncovered in this book have revealed one of the mechanisms behind social stratification. That is, we have shown one way in which families' biological legacies and economic legacies are replicated across generations and over time. As low-birth-weight-and-low-income parents pass on to their children their birth weight and their economic status, they are increasing the chances that their children will find themselves in similar biological and economic situations.

On the policy side, we have made various suggestions of how social programs may intervene in these ongoing cycles. With regard to preventing low birth weight, we have made two proposals. When possible and appropriate under existing policy guidelines, family histories of low birth weight should be taken into account in eligibility and benefit-level criteria. Alternatively, when such biological specificity is not appropriate, we have suggested that pregnancies should be considered "qualifying events" that raise the income eligibility criteria of various social programs. With respect to reducing the negative consequences associated with low birth weight, we have made additional proposals. We have suggested that, as children proceed through their educational careers, low-birth-weight status ought to be noted in the diagnosis and treatment of disabilities. Attention to birth weight status may help parents, teachers, and physicians recognize and refine treatments for disability and developmental delay.

Turning from the level of state and federal policy, there also appears to be a place for attention to biosocial risk at the individual level. It seems that biological and social risk factors could also be considered in certain physician-patient relationships. Family histories and individual medical histories already play an important role in medicine in assessing individuals' risks for particular diseases and disabilities. Thus we would simply suggest that questions about parental birth weight (mother's and father's birth weights alike) ought to be standard when physicians take medical histories of pregnant women. Based on an informal and anecdotal survey of obstetricians, we found that, at this time, such questions about the birth weight or premature status of parents are not part of standard risk assessments of pregnant women. However, such attention to familial risk of low birth weight could allow physicians and mothers alike to pay extra attention to, and possibly to improve, clinical issues associated with birth weight, such as maternal weight gain, early labor, and rates of fetal growth.

Data, Variables, and Methods

DATA

We use the two following data sets in our analyses:

Panel Study of Income Dynamics (PSID)

The PSID is a nationally representative, longitudinal sample of American families who were first interviewed in 1968. The PSID initially surveyed a total of 4,800 families and consisted of two independent samples: a broadly representative, cross-sectional national sample, supplemented by a more focused, national sample of low-income families. The PSID has grown since its inception as it follows new households that have formed out of the original 4,800. Among those tracked are the children in the initial sample and those subsequently born or moved into a sample household. As a result of its success in following young adults as they form their own families, the PSID includes more than 7,000 families as of 2001.[1]

In chapter 2, when considering differences in the heritability of low birth weight by race, we draw from the PSID a subsample that includes individuals whose mothers were sample members in addition and who have valid responses on both their own and their parent's birth weight indicators (as well as on the other variables in the analysis). For this group, we chose to use the original family sampling weight from 1968, the first year of the survey (though use of the latest, individual-level weight does not alter results). Finally, we restrict our subsample for this analysis to whites and blacks only who were singleton births. See Table 2.1 in appendix B for descriptive statistics pertaining to this subsample.

In chapter 3, when considering the risk of low birth weight, we use a sub-sample of the PSID that includes children born between 1986 and 1992 for whom birth weight information is available and whose mothers were in the sample during their pregnancy. See appendix B, Table 3.1, for descriptive statistics pertaining to this sample and Table 3.2 for various subsample comparisons relevant to this analysis of low birth weight. In chapter 4, when considering the relationship between low birth weight and educational attainment, we use a PSID subsample that includes only those individuals who had reached their 19th birthday by the end of 1992 and who had a valid indicator of birth weight status. A description of this sample can be found in appendix B, Table 4.1, and further subsample comparisons relevant to this analysis of educational attainment can be found in Table 4.2.

1995–1997 Matched Multiple Birth Data Set

The Matched Multiple Birth Data Set was developed to allow for the analysis of births and infant deaths in multiple deliveries. This data set was created by combining the restricted-use U.S. Live Birth and Fetal Death files for 1995–1997 (a data set maintained by the National Center for Health Statistics) with the Linked Live Birth/Infant Death Cohort Data Sets for 1995–1997 (another data set maintained by the National Center for Health Statistics in which information from birth certificates is matched with information from death certificates). Members of twin and triplet birth sets were first identified by matching records within the U.S. Live Birth and Fetal Death files for 1995–1997. This file of multiple birth sets was then matched with the Linked Live Birth/Infant Death Cohort Data Sets for 1995–1997 in order to identify infant deaths that corresponded to the live twin and triplet birth records.[2] The total number of matched cases that emerged from this effort was 320,534.[3] In our analysis of infant mortality, we are concerned only with twin pairs that have valid information on all of our variables. This yields a total sample size of 265,370. For descriptive statistics of this sample, by discordancy and sex, see Table 4.5 in appendix B.

While the Matched Multiple Birth Data Set contains several variables ranging from number of prenatal visits to specific causes of death, it does not have data on zygosity, that is, whether twin pairs are identical or fraternal. We are able to deduce this information, however, by breaking down our sample by sex. We know that all mixed-sex twin pairs are fraternal. We further know, based on national averages, that 50 percent of same sex twins are identical. And this rate is the same for boys and girls, so that 50 percent of all boy twin pairs will be identical and 50 percent of all girl twin pairs will be identical. In our analysis we find no significant interactions between birth weight and sex.[4] In the mixed-sex subsample the interaction term for birth weight by sex is not statistically significant, and we further find no difference in birth weight parameters across our all-boy or all-girl subsamples. This lack of an interaction between birth weight and sex allows us to assume that differences in birth weight parameters between our same-sex and mixed-sex subsamples are not due to sex differences but rather to differences in zygosity. This assumption about genetic variation then allows us to sort out "true" birth weight effects from situations in which birth weight effects are a proxy for alternative underlying health conditions.

Another way to consider this deduction of zygosity is to note that if:

a = effect of birth weight for fraternals
b = effect of weight for identicals (what we are trying to pin down)
c = effect of weight for boys' (or girls') group
p = the fraction of identical twins in the boys' (or girls') group

then we can treat c as a weighted average of a and b:

$$c = bp + a\,(1-p)$$

Since we know c, a, and p, we can solve for b:

$$b = \frac{c - a(1-p)}{p}$$

VARIABLES

We use the following variables in our analyses:

Birth Weight

This key variable serves as both a predictor and an outcome measure in this book. While for children born between 1986 and 1992 the PSID inquired into their exact birth weight in ounces, for sample members who were born prior to 1986 only a binary variable is available indicating whether or not an individual weighed less than 2,500 grams at birth. If the individual weighed less than this amount, then he or she received a score of one on this indicator; otherwise, the variable was scored as a zero. In chapter 2, when examining how the inheritance of low birth weight varies by race, we use this dummy variable to indicate both parental and filial low-birth-weight status. In chapter 3, when comparing the effects of parental low birth weight and income on the risk of filial low birth weight, we use this dichotomous variable to indicate parental low-birth-weight status but use actual birth weight measured in ounces for the filial outcome measure. In chapter 4, when examining the effect of birth weight on educational attainment, we again use the actual birth weight measure (in ounces), this time as an independent variable rather than an outcome. Finally, in chapter 4, when examining the relationship between birth weight and infant morality, we draw our data not from the PSID but from the Matched Multiple Birth file. Thus, in this case, birth weight is a continuous variable measured in pounds.[5]

Sex

Research has shown that the entire birth weight distribution of females is shifted to the left of that of males, and thus females have a greater risk of being born low birth weight than males.[6] However (perhaps because of the shift in the female birth weight distribution), low-birth-weight females have been shown to suffer fewer of the health and developmental problems associated with low birth weight.[7] Factoring out the respondent's sex is, therefore, important to all of the models in this book. This variable is used to control for differential risk of low birth weight in chapters 2 and 3 when we are treating low birth weight as an outcome. However, this variable is also used to control for differential risk of infant mortality and untimely high school graduation when, alternatively, we are treating low birth weight as an independent variable. Because low birth weight may pose less of a health risk to female infants than to male infants, its role in infant mortality may vary depending on sex. In the educational analysis, such a control is also necessary. Partly because low birth weight may have different long-term implications for males compared to females and partly because females in general have been shown to attain higher levels of education than their male counterparts, the respondent's sex may further confound estimates of birth weight effects in this analysis as well.[8]

Birth Order

Depending on whether we are analyzing twins or singleton births, this variable may indicate considerably different situations. Because research has shown that firstborns may be at higher risk of low birth weight, in cases of singleton births, a dummy variable was constructed to indicate whether the individual was the first child born to his or her mother.[9] For the prediction of educational attainment, this term was also included, because researchers have shown that children who come from smaller families and those who are firstborn tend to do better educationally than those from large families and those who are of higher birth order.[10]

Firstborn children may face a higher risk of low birth weight for biological reasons. The placenta forms as an "immunological" barrier between the mother and the "foreign" body (i.e., the fetus) that occupies her uterus. The stronger the immune response, the bigger the placenta that develops and the lower risk for low birth weight. Here we are dealing with a process comparable to animistic response. Specifically, when a person is exposed to the same antigens more than once, the immune reaction is swifter and more complete. That is, when the body has been exposed to a particular antigen previously, it already has a "blueprint" for its responses and thus has a faster, more complete reaction.[11] According to this logic, second- and higher-order births should benefit from previous pregnancies through the development of stronger, larger placentas.

However, such biological risk factors in first births are also likely taking place in the midst of several social risk factors as well. Firstborns are more likely to be unintended (mistimed, unwanted, or both) than second borns.[12] The possible shock and depression accompanying the discovery of an unwanted pregnancy may have a negative impact on the outcome of the pregnancy. Also, if the woman was not aware of being pregnant initially, she may continue to drink or smoke further into the gestation period. However, while pregnancy wantedness has been shown to have a positive effect on behaviors that increase birth weight (i.e., early prenatal care and maternal weight gain), it has not been shown to determine the risk of low birth weight.[13] Another possible reason that firstborns face a higher risk of low birth weight may have to do with the parental learning process. Parents may be more likely to make "mistakes" the first time around—that is, smoking, drinking, or not initiating prenatal care early enough, for instance. These behavioral differences—independent of pregnancy intentionality status—could generate a higher risk for firstborns. Additionally, these behavioral factors may be compounded by economic risk factors. Evidence suggests that family income and wealth tend to increase over time so that firstborn children are more likely to be born into a socioeconomically disadvantaged family.

In cases when we are analyzing twin births, this variable does not imply that the individual was the first child born to his or her mother but rather means that the individual was the first child born *within the twin set*. In this analysis, it is possible that a mother had births prior to the multiple birth set in question. Regardless, we still call the first twin to be born in this birth set the "firstborn." It is necessary to control for such firstborn status in multiple birth sets because evidence suggests that second-born twins are at higher risk than firstborn twins for various health complications and for neonatal mortality.[14]

Mother's Age

The literature has shown that children born to mothers who are under age 18 or over 34 are more likely to be born low birth weight.[15] Further, evidence suggests that children born to young mothers may face educational risk. Therefore, we use dummy variables for both young maternal age and advanced maternal age in our analyses of the risk of low birth weight; however, we use only a single dummy variable for young maternal age in our analysis of the risk of "late" high school graduation.

There is a fair amount of debate over the mechanisms that account for the effects of young maternal age on birth weight. Some authors have suggested that age affects low birth weight through biological pathways. For instance, researchers have suggested that fetuses in pregnancies in young women may be undernourished because the mother is still growing and thus requires nutrients that would be going to the fetus if the woman were older.[16] Many other authors, however, have suggested that the disadvantaged social position of most pregnant teens may account for the effects of young maternal age on birth weight. The decision to bear children early is intimately linked to socioeconomic status and future prospects, such that poor teenagers with few prospects for higher education or employment are much more likely to bear children.[17] The effects of age on birth weight may thus be a result of the fact that young mothers are much more likely than older mothers to be disadvantaged.

Maternal age may additionally matter in the long-term educational outcomes of low birth weight children. Children born to young mothers tend to demonstrate lower levels of educational achievement and attainment,[18] and thus a low-birth-weight baby born to a young mother may face greater risk than other low-birth-weight children (advanced maternal age was not a factor among this second PSID subsample and is therefore not presented). As was the case above, however, some researchers, such as Arline Geronimus and her colleagues, argue that the effects of young maternal age on intellectual developmental measures are an artifact of unobserved socioeconomic family differences, such as income or environment. Using cousin comparisons to factor out between-family variations, these authors find that maternal age at time of birth has no effect on later outcomes.[19] The within-family comparisons we employ in this book similarly factor out such unobserved variation in the effects of maternal age, and thus any variation in educational attainment attributable to maternal age in this analysis will likely represent a true effect.

Marital Status

In addition to maternal age, we include in our analyses of low birth weight and educational attainment an indicator of whether the mother was married at the time of the individual's birth. This is by no means a perfect indicator of the absence of an adult partner, since unmarried women may be in a cohabiting union or living with family members. However, mothers who are not married during their pregnancies are more likely to spend a significant amount of time without the social or financial support of a partner than those who live in a married, two-parent household. This lack of support may influence birth outcomes by increasing stress and social isolation or by further disadvantaging an already at-risk woman. Indeed, single status has been shown to exacerbate various inequalities associated with birth weight. For instance, researchers have documented a significant difference in birth weight by race for unmarried women but have found no such racial variation for married women. These researchers similarly found that differential access to health care, specifically prenatal care, affected low birth weight for unmarried women but not for married women.[20] The financial and social support associated with marital status may thus reduce some of the impact of the inequalities that are related to birth weight patterns.

Mother's marital status at the time of birth may similarly affect children's long-term success and thus is included in our analysis of educational attainment as well. In our analyses of education, we will be unable to consider whether the mother marries at some point after the birth of the child. This, however, is not cause for very great concern since evidence suggests that prenatal and early childhood conditions are very important in determining individuals' long-term outcomes. The lack of social and financial support associated with single motherhood even at the beginning of the child's life can have lasting effects—indeed, family structure as early as age two has been shown to affect test scores.[21]

Maternal Education

Maternal education is a very important variable in our efforts to control for socioeconomic conditions. It is, therefore, included in our models of the risk of low birth weight, as well as in our models of the risk of low educational attainment. One of the strongest socioeconomic predictors of rates of low birth weight is maternal education. Maternal education itself is possibly a result of both genetic and environmental conditions, and thus it is important to control for this measure when estimating the effects of heredity of low birth weight. The possible genetic component of maternal education would also be important in our analysis of educational outcomes because an innate intelligence or academic ability may be passed on from mother to child and may influence the child's later educational attainment. However, if there is such a genetic component to educational attainment, it is not separate from environment or behavior. Education is strongly linked to greater health knowledge and more healthful behaviors and may thereby reduce the risk of low birth weight.[22] Additionally, a higher level of maternal education may foster child development via behavior and thus may have a positive nonbiological/nongenetic effect on children's later educational attainment. More educated mothers are more likely to buy educational toys for and engage in educational activities with children, both of which have been shown to have positive effects on children's academic achievement. More educated mothers are also more likely to understand child development and therefore may be better at assisting their children's progress than less educated mothers.[23]

This relationship between maternal education and home environment is likely to be particularly important for low-birth-weight children, and maternal education may indeed be a crucial nonbiological mechanism driving the association between low birth weight and low academic achievement. Since the majority of low-birth-weight children are born to mothers with little education and low incomes, it follows that these children are in early childhood environments that may not foster their development. It is therefore possible that maternal education and the environmental factors associated with it may be, at least partially, to blame for low-birth-weight children's low educational attainment. Factoring maternal education out of our analyses will thus allow us to more effectively capture true health effects in low birth weight and educational attainment.

Race

There is considerable variation in rates of low birth weight and levels of educational attainment across several racial and ethnic groups in the United States. However, in our analyses we choose to compare only African Americans to all other racial and ethnic groups, because African Americans' risks for low birth weight and low educational attainment are notably higher than those of other racial/ethnic groups. Indeed, rates of low birth weight among blacks are almost twice as high as rates for most other groups in the United States.[24] Researchers have very little understanding of or consensus on why this difference is so large. Factoring out socioeconomic differences between blacks and whites generally significantly reduces, but does not eliminate, the differences in black and white rates of low birth weight.[25] That is, in almost all analyses, there remains racial variation in low birth weight that is not attributable to socioeconomic differences. Several authors have argued that this remaining variation could be the results of genetic differences between African Americans and whites, and we outline in chapter 2 the very mixed results that surround such claims.

African Americans are further generally found to be at a rather stark disad-vantage in terms of educational attainment (although this disadvantage is gen-erally stronger for African American men than for African American women).[26] Again, there is very little consensus on the mechanisms behind this difference. As with birth weight, there is debate as to whether educational disadvantages can be attributed to socioeconomic differences between blacks and whites or to more subtle aspects of race. In general evidence surrounding this debate, which is reviewed in some detail in chapter 2, is quite mixed.

Income-to-Needs Ratio

This variable is constructed by dividing the total family income for a given year by the poverty threshold for the family's size as determined by the U.S. Depart-ment of Agriculture and the U.S. Census Bureau. This "Orshansky ratio" is expressed as a "percentage of poverty" such that a value less than 1.0 means that the respondent's family lived in poverty for the given year.[27] Total family income includes all forms of cash, including that received from labor market earnings by any member of the family unit, informal gifts, investment income, and government transfers. In-kind benefits (such as Food Stamps) are not included, however. The time period we consider in the birth weight analysis is the year prior to birth and thus includes the mother's pregnancy and the period immediately preceding it.[28] In the educational models, we use income in the first five years of life. Overwhelmingly, evidence suggests that early childhood poverty has lasting effects on ability and achievement.[29]

While many researchers agree that income poverty is an important factor in both birth weight and educational attainment, the subtleties of its effects and mechanisms remain subjects of debate. For instance, it is not clear that income has universal effects on birth weight across racial and ethnic groups.[30] While some researchers have found that the effects of poverty on low birth weight vary by race and ethnicity, others have found no such variation. The mecha-nisms through which poverty affects birth weight also remain unclear. Many scholars suggest that poverty affects birth weight via biological pathways, such as nutritional deficits,[31] while others suggest that poverty affects birth weight through behavioral and social pathways, such as poor women's lower rates of prenatal care and higher rates of smoking.[32] How early childhood poverty may affect later achievement is similarly debated. Since socioeconomic conditions in early childhood have been shown to have lasting effects on health and cognitive ability, socioeconomic status may affect educational attainment through bio-logical pathways. For instance, childhood poverty may lead to poor health, which in turn leads to missing many days of school. Or cognitive deficiencies resulting from childhood or prenatal poverty may cause children to be held back a grade.[33] Growing up in poverty, however, also has very strong effects on children's aspirations and mental well-being, and thus home environment may also shape educational achievement through nonbiological pathways.[34] For instance, when living in a poor neighborhood that offers few job opportunities, children may have difficulty recognizing the benefits of education and, therefore, may have low aspirations that lead to dropping out. We explore these possible biological and social mechanisms in greater detail in chapter 4.

We should note that in our analyses of timely high school graduation, we estimated the models with various functional forms of the income-to-needs ratio. These included the logged ratio and various categorical specifications, such as under 50 percent of the poverty threshold, 50 to 100 percent of the threshold, and so on. The results (specifically, the insignificance of the main income effect) were not sensitive to the functional form adopted.

High School Graduation

For the analyses of the effect of low birth weight on educational attainment, our main outcome variable is completion of high school "on time"—that is, by one's 19th birthday. Graduating on time is substantively important with respect to the life chances of young adults. Those who graduate "late" are more likely to have received a high school equivalency diploma (GED) than those who finished their secondary schooling "on time."[35] An equivalency diploma, in turn, results in poorer economic outcomes—as measured by hours worked or wages—when contrasted to the results of actual high school attendance.[36] Also, students who do not complete high school "on time" are less likely to attend four-year academic colleges if they continue their educational careers than are "traditional" students.[37] Timely high school graduation, then, is strongly related to adult socioeconomic status.

This association between low income and high school graduation further allows us to consider cycles of socioeconomic status across generations and address how health may be affecting these cycles. If a low-birth-weight baby is born into poverty (as indicated by maternal income both during pregnancy and during the first five years of life) and does not graduate from high school by age 19, likely leading to poorer adult economic outcomes, we find an intergenerational cycle of poverty that can be considered in conjunction with an intergenerational cycle of birth weight (as indicated by parental and filial birth weight measures).

Repeating a Grade, Special Education, Learning Impairment

In order to test the robustness of the effect of low birth weight on educational attainment, we employ three additional measures of educational progress. The first of these measures is a dummy variable indicating whether an individual ever repeated a grade. This variable is based the following question from the 1995 PSID: "Since starting kindergarten, has (the respondent) ever repeated a grade or been held back because the school recommended it?"[38] Approximately 10 percent of our sample was held back a grade at some point in their educational careers. As we discussed in chapter 4, with the above measure of timely high school graduation, it is possible that one may graduate "late" not because of slow or problematic educational progress but because of entering school late. This possibility may be particularly likely for low-birth-weight or premature children, who may begin kindergarten later than normal-birth-weight, full-term children because of poor health or gestational age. Considering this additional outcome of being held back a grade will give us a sense of the extent to which "late" graduation among low-birth-weight children is the result of educational problems or simply a delay in beginning education.

The second additional educational outcome that we employ is a dummy variable indicating whether the respondent has ever been in a special educational program. This variable is based the question from the 1995 PSID, "Has (the respondent) ever been classified by the school as needing special education?"[39] About 5.5 percent of the children in our sample had at some point participated in a special education program. The third additional educational outcome that we employ is a dummy variable indicating whether the respondent was ever categorized as learning impaired. This variable is based on the question from the same year of the PSID, "Has (the respondent) ever been classified as learning disabled, perceptually impaired or speech impaired?"[40] Again, about 5.5 percent of our sample was at some point treated as learning impaired. Both of these further educational variables, like the first variable measuring grade repetition, should allow us not only to assess the robustness of our low birth weight estimates but also to obtain a more detailed picture of how low-birth-weight children may be "held up" in their educational progress.

Infant Mortality, Neonatal Mortality, Postneonatal Mortality

When estimating the effects of birth weight on infant mortality in our twin analyses, we use three different measures of mortality. First, we use overall infant mortality, defined as death under one year of age, as an outcome measure. However, we also decompose this measure into neonatal mortality (death under 28 days of age) and postneonatal mortality (between 28 days and one year) as subsequent outcome measures.[41] Breaking down measures of infant mortality in this way is necessary because striking differences are apparent when comparing causes of death in the neonatal and postneonatal periods. Disorders related to short gestation and low birth weight are the primary cause of neonatal infant death, while sudden infant death syndrome is the primary cause of postneonatal infant death.[42] Since we are concerned in this twin analysis with the precise effect of birth weight on infant mortality, attention to this difference between the neonatal and postneonatal periods will be particularly important.

THE WITHIN-FAMILY COMPARISON APPROACH

The within-family comparison approach (also known as fixed-effects models) represents an effective way of factoring out unobserved differences between respondents that may be generating biased effects in standard regression models. As mentioned in chapter 1, it may not be the effect of income per se that generates a significant coefficient with respect to some health or socioeconomic outcome but rather the unobserved characteristics of those who tend to have high or low incomes. By contrasting individuals from the same family of origin, we eliminate most of the potentially biasing factors. These include genetic endowments, permanent income (expected lifetime earnings), and social class more generally (to the extent that it is shared by family members). In short, anything that is shared by family members is factored out. So the effect of income, for instance, is only the effect of the transient portion of income, the difference between two time periods (in the case of the birth weight analysis, years between two pregnancies). As such, fixed-effects coefficients represent lower-bound estimates of the "true" effect. However, any effect that is presented as significant in this framework has passed a very strict test, immune to most concerns of unobserved variable bias, to the extent that these results are from across-family factors. There still remains the possibility that spurious effects may appear due to associations of within-family differences. Once again, fixed-effects models cannot incorporate the notion of interbirth changes in behavior with respect to those behaviors about which we have no data. We cannot address, for example, the possibility that changes in prenatal care took place from one birth to the next.

The fixed-effects approach differs from ordinary least-squares approaches and so merits some elaboration here. The traditional ordinary least-squares formulation is expressed in the equation:

$$Y = \alpha + X\beta + \varepsilon, \tag{1}$$

where X represents the matrix of variables and observations specified in the model and β represents its associated vector of coefficients. However, in the case of low birth weight and educational progress, for example, we can be fairly certain there are lurking variables—that is, that there is another matrix of unobserved characteristics that is biasing our estimates of β. As discussed in chapters 1 through 4, a whole host of unobserved characteristics affect both filial birth weight and parental socioeconomic circumstances (or filial educational attainment and parental socioeconomic circumstances).

With this in mind, as shown in equation 2, we can explicitly incorporate such unobserved characteristics into a model. In our case, they break out into two parts: the unobserved factors that are common to families and those that are unique to individuals.

$$Y = \alpha + X\beta + FAM\gamma + IND\delta + \varepsilon' \tag{2}$$

Now we have made explicit the problem of the correlation between these unobserved sets of variables, FAM and IND, and our observed set of variables. When we have panel data, we can solve this problem, as shown in equation 3, by taking difference scores between our Y variable (say birth weight) at times t_1 and t_2 and regressing that against the difference in X variables (say income) at times t_1 and t_2.[43] In this equation, the unobserved family-level characteristics that are assumed to remain constant over time drop out in modeling the difference:

$$\Delta Y_{t_1,t_2} = \alpha + \Delta X_{t_1,t_2}\beta + \Delta IND_{t_1,t_2}\delta + \Delta\varepsilon'_{t_1,t_2} \tag{3}$$

In our case, however, times t_1 and t_2 actually represent the birth years of different, nontwin siblings. Thus, we have not eliminated unobserved characteristics that are unique to the individual siblings. For example, we cannot eliminate bias in our models that may be due to the fact that a mother smoked during one pregnancy and not during another, gained a lot of weight during one pregnancy and not during another, sought differing levels of prenatal care for the two pregnancies, or used alcohol during one and not during another. These are individual unobserved differences. To the extent that these differences are correlated with our X variables, β will be biased. For example, to the extent that drinking or drug use during pregnancy (or in between pregnancies 1 and 2) caused the mother's income to drop or her marital status to change, we would be overestimating the effect of these variables in our equations. However, to the extent that our X variables are causally prior to these unobserved, individual-level characteristics, their omission is not as troubling but merely suggests that part of the effects we report may work indirectly through such mechanisms (i.e., weight gain or prenatal care access).

One additional note: we do not restrict our analysis to sibling pairs but rather allow varying numbers of siblings for each family. So our technique is not as straightforward as regressing a difference score. Rather, the fixed-effects models we employ essentially regress the score on the Y variable against the scores on the vector of X variables while including indicator variables for all families save one (this is done implicitly by the STATA software). This is equivalent to taking out the mean value for each family of siblings (and losing a degree of freedom for each in the process). So for example, in our fixed-effects model of high school graduation, we have 1,388 valid responses of individuals from a total of 766 family units. We lose a degree of freedom for taking out the mean of 765 of those family units (one is the suppressed category on mother's ID). It is conceptually equivalent to the two-sibling model, where by calculating the difference in their scores, the sample size shifts from 1,000 individuals to 500 pairs.

INTERPRETING THE EFFECTS

In many of the figures in this book, we display the impact of a certain characteristic on a particular outcome variable. For example, in Table 2.3 (appendix B) and Figure 2.4 we explore the influence of race on the risk of a baby being born low birth weight. The coefficients shown in the table allow us to judge whether a variable is significant—that is, whether that characteristic bears a meaningful relationship to the risk of low birth weight. However precise the coefficient may be, it is difficult to interpret just how large an influence that variable wields on low birth weight. Thus, in order to facilitate the interpretation of these effects, we translate the coefficients in the various models given in Table 2.3 into straightforward percentage increases (or decreases) in the risk of having a low-birth-weight child as a result of the mother being African American.

In Table 2.3, the risk of low birth weight is expressed as a "log-odds ratio." The term *ratio* refers simply to the ratio of the probability p that a baby with a set of attributes (personal, parental, environmental, etc.) will be born low birth weight to its complement, $1 - p$. We take the natural logarithm of the ratio to form our dependent variable. The equation representing Model 1—the basic bivariate model, in which we have just one independent variable (African

American) and the dependent variable (the log-odds of being born low birth weight)—is as follows:

$$\log \frac{p}{1-p} = \beta_0 + \beta_1 AfricanAmerican$$

The variable *AfricanAmerican* assumes the value of one if the child is African American and zero if not. Our objective is to solve for *p*—the probability that a baby is born low birth weight—under each of two conditions: African American and non–African American. By way of minor algebraic manipulation, we find that

$$p = \frac{\exp[\beta_0 + \beta_1 \, AfricanAmerican]}{1 + \exp[\beta_0 + \beta_1 \, AfricanAmerican]}$$

where *exp* refers to the exponentiation of whatever is within brackets. For African American babies, then, *AfricanAmerican* equals one, and

$$p_{AfAm} = \frac{\exp[\beta_0 + \beta_1]}{1 + \exp[\beta_0 + \beta_1]}$$

For babies who are not African American,

$$p_{notAfAm} = \frac{\exp[\beta_0]}{1 + \exp[\beta_0]}$$

Plugging in the values of the coefficients β_0 and β_1, we have $p_{AfAm} = .091$ and $p_{notAfAm} = .044$. The percentage additional risk in being born low birth weight that is associated with African American babies versus non–African American babies is $100 \times [(p_{AfAm}/p_{not\text{-}AfAm}) - 1]$ or $100 \times (2.09 - 1)$, which is 109 percent.

The complete model, Model E in Table 2.3 is somewhat more complex to understand. Here, the equation fully spelled out is:

$$\log \frac{p}{1-p} = \beta_0 + \beta_1 Female + \beta_2 FirstBorn + \beta_3 AfricanAmerican$$
$$+ \beta_4 Income\text{-}to\text{-}Needs + \beta_5 MomEducation + \beta_6 MomMarried$$
$$+ \beta_7 MomUnder18 + \beta_8 MomLBW + \beta_9 DadLBW$$

In this instance, we want to determine the impact of being African American on low birth weight while at the same time controlling for the influence of many other variables. For all factors other than race, we substitute the mean value of each variable and then multiply it by the coefficient associated with that variable. African American, once again, takes on the value of either zero or one. The equation thus reads:

$$\log \frac{p}{1-p} = \beta_0 + \beta_1 \overline{Female} + \beta_2 \overline{FirstBorn} + \beta_3 AfricanAmerican$$
$$+ \beta_4 \overline{Income\text{-}to\text{-}Needs} + \beta_5 \overline{MomEducation} + \beta_6 \overline{MomMarried}$$
$$+ \beta_7 \overline{MomUnder18} + \beta_8 \overline{MomLBW} + \beta_9 \overline{DadLBW}$$

All mean values can be obtained from Table 2.1 (appendix B) in the first column, where we see that the sample size is 4,431 (the same sample used for the models estimated in Table 2.3). The mean values for the continuous variables, such as the income-to-needs ratio (2.914) or maternal education (12.594), are obvious. However, the mean values of the dichotomous variables, such as mother low birth weight (.071) or female child (.480), are simply the proportion having that characteristic. The log-odds ratio, then, is equal to:

$$\log \frac{p}{1-p} = -3.232 + .442(.480) + .169(.337) + .348(0/1)$$
$$+.006(2.914) - .072(12.594) + .105(.920)$$
$$+.320(.012) + 2.063(.071) + 2.722(.054)$$

which is −3.11 for African Americans and −3.46 for those who are not African American. Transforming these log-odds ratios, we find that for these two groups the probabilities of being born low birth weight, p, are .043 and .031.

The rise in the likelihood of being born low birth weight that is due to being African American is 40 percent, that is, $100 \times [(.043/.031)-1]$. The most important fact to note in Table 2.3, as we shift from Model A to Model E, is that the coefficient of the African American variable diminishes considerably, cut by more than half from .790 to .348. The bottom line effect of race shown in Figure 2.4 declines concomitantly, from 109 percent to 40 percent. The reason for this reduction is that new factors in Model E have been allowed—by virtue of incorporating them in the model—to account for some of the variation in low-birth-weight status among infants. By comparing the full and bivariate models, we find that some of the *apparent* impact of race can be explained by variations in other variables that are correlated with race. For example, lower educational attainment is associated with higher rates of low birth weight, and at the same time, African Americans are found to have lower average levels of education than non–African Americans. Consequently, when we do not include education in our model, we are falsely attributing the negative effect of education on low birth weight to African American status. Thus, the coefficient for African American exaggerates the effect of being African American on low birth weight. When we incorporate the mother's educational attainment in our model, we are able to estimate the "pure" effect of race on low-birth-weight status *independent* of the mother's educational status. In the full model, we are able to discount appropriately for a range of factors in addition to educational attainment.

In a variation of this approach, we assess the impact of income on the likelihood of graduating high school in a timely fashion, that is, by one's 19th birthday. We operationalize income as a family's income-to-needs ratio, which is simply the ratio of a family's income to the poverty threshold designated by the federal government for a family of that size. The poverty line for a family of four in 2001 was $18,103. For example, the income-to-needs ratio for a family of four with an income of $27,000 is approximately 1.5 ($27,000/$18,103).

In the last bar of Figure 4.1, we graph the increase in the probability of "timely" graduation from high school that is due to a rise in the income-to-needs ratio of one unit (or by $18,103, in the previous example).

To obtain the last bar in Figure 4.1, we have applied the model estimated in the third column of Table 4.3 in appendix B. Here we focus on a child who was born low birth weight; thus that variable has a value of one. The interaction variable—between low birth weight and the income-to-needs ratio—also applies because we are estimating the effect for a low-birth-weight child. All variables are given their mean values, as in the previous examples. To judge the impact of a unit increase in the income-to-needs ratio, we choose the unit change to occur about the mean of the income-to-needs ratio variable, which is 3.303 (see Table 4.1, appendix B). Consequently, we substitute a value of 3.303 ± 0.5—or, 2.803 and 3.803—for the income-to-needs ratio variable, in addition to all of the other variable means. We find that $p_{\text{income-to-needs} = 2.803} =$ .3128 and that $p_{\text{income-to-needs} = 3.803} = .4005$, implying that a one-unit increase in the income-to-needs ratio about the mean results in a 28 percent increase (i.e., $100 \times [(.4005/.3128) - 1]$) in the probability of graduating from high school in a timely fashion. This estimated increase is net of the potentially confounding influences recognized in the model.

Tables

TABLE 2.1. DESCRIPTIVE STATISTICS FOR
ANALYSES OF LOW BIRTH WEIGHT, BY RACE

Variable	Total	Blacks	Whites & Others
Filial low birth rate	.057	.091	.044
	(.232)	(.288)	(.204)
	[19.30%]	[28.35%]	[15.60%]
Female child	.480	.472	.483
	(.500)	(.500)	(.500)
	[77.93%]	[78.12%]	[77.85%]
Firstborn status	.337	.291	.356
	(.473)	(.454)	(.479)
	[86.89%]	[80.76%]	[89.39%]
African American race	.290	—	—
	(.454)		
	[00.00%]		
Income-to-needs ratio			
year prior to birth	2.914	2.050	3.266
	(2.082)	(1.460)	(2.193)
[Std. dev. between group]	[1.862]	[1.428]	[1.906]
[Std. dev. within group]	[1.180]	[.844]	[1.292]
Mother under 18			
at birth of child	.012	.022	.008
	(.110)	(.149)	(.089)
	[5.87%]	[10.12%]	[4.13%]
Mother married			
at birth of child	.920	.792	.973
	(.270)	(.406)	(.162)
	[19.12%]	[42.29%]	[9.66%]
Maternal education			
(highest grade			
completed [HGC])	12.594	11.920	12.868
	(2.200)	(2.060)	(2.197)
[Std. dev. between group]	[2.090]	[2.005]	[2.056]
[Std. dev. within group]	[.957]	[.978]	[.949]
Mother low birth weight	.071	.116	.052
	(.256)	(.320)	(.222)
	[10.24%]	[11.84%]	[6.44%]
Father low birth weight	.054	.088	.040
	(.225)	(.283)	(.195)
	[6.50%]	[9.34%]	[5.34%]
N	4,431	1,284	3,147

NOTE: Mean values shown, with standard deviations in parentheses and percentage discordant within families in brackets.

TABLE 2.2. ZERO ORDER CORRELATIONS FOR VARIABLES INCLUDED
IN ANALYSIS OF RACE EFFECTS ON LOW BIRTH WEIGHT ($N = 4,431$)

Variable	(1)	(2)	(3)	(4)	(5)	(6)	(7)	(8)	(9)	(10)
Dependent Variable										
Filial low birth weight	1.000	—	—	—	—	—	—	—	—	—
Independent Variables										
Female child	.037*	1.000	—	—	—	—	—	—	—	—
Firstborn status	.005	-.009	1.000	—	—	—	—	—	—	—
African American race	.093***	-.010	-.062***	1.000	—	—	—	—	—	—
Income-to-needs ratio, year prior to death	-.040**	.003	.052***	-.265***	1.000	—	—	—	—	—
Mother under 18 at child's birth	.008	.005	.151***	.061***	-.075***	1.000	—	—	—	—
Mother married at child's birth	-.053***	-.014	-.082***	-.304***	.196***	-.173***	1.000	—	—	—
Maternal education (HGC by 1984)	-.053***	-.011	.085***	-.195***	.454***	-.093***	.161***	1.000	—	—
Mother low birth weight	.315***	.005	-.007	.113***	-.027+	-.015	-.079***	-.032*	1.000	—
Father low birth weight	.398***	.000	-.011	.097***	-.040**	-.008	-.060***	-.038*	.223***	1.000

***$p < .001$ **$p < .01$ *$p < .05$ +$p < .10$ (two-tailed tests)

TABLE 2.3. EFFECT OF RACE ON RISK OF FILIAL LOW
BIRTH WEIGHT, LOGISTIC REGRESSION MODELS

Variable	Model A	Model B	Model C	Model D	Model E
Respondent Characteristics					
Female child		.316* [2.409]	.326* [2.480]		.442** [2.919]
Firstborn status		.062 [.132]	.117 [.876]		.169 [1.036]
African American race	.790*** [5.201]		.694*** [4.101]	.354* [2.156]	.348* [1.993]
Socioeconomic Variables					
Income-to-needs ratio, year prior to birth		-.038 [-.919]	-.001 [-.038]		.006 [.145]
Mother's education (HGC by 1984)		-.076* [-2.261]	-.070* [-2.025]		-.072 [-.929]
Mother married at child's birth		-.515* [-2.318]	-.229 [-.976]		.105 [.336]
Mother under 18 at child's birth		-.196 [-.351]	-.215 [-.373]		.320 [.520]
Parental Characteristics					
Mother low birth weight				2.051*** [10.747]	2.063*** [10.686]
Father low birth weight				2.698*** [14.537]	2.722*** [14.537]
Constant	-3.090*** [-31.450]	-1.468*** [-3.674]	-2.186*** [-4.722]	-3.715*** [-33.768]	-3.232*** [-6.692]
L^2_{df}	27.05_1	23.92_6	45.96_7	322.57_3	328.55_9
N	4,431	4,431	4,431	4,431	4,431

NOTE: Standard errors robust to clustering within families. Long-odds ratios shown, with t-statistics in brackets.

***$p < .001$ **$p < .01$ *$p < .05$

TABLE 2.4. EFFECT OF PARENTAL LOW BIRTH
WEIGHT AND SOCIOECONOMIC CONDITIONS
ON RISK OF FILIAL LOW BIRTH WEIGHT,
BY RACE—LOGISTIC REGRESSION MODELS

Variable	Blacks Only[a]	Whites & Others Only
Respondent Characteristics		
Female child	.213	.633**
	[.952]	[3.048]
Firstborn status	.262	.087
	[1.027]	[.413]
Socioeconomic Variables:		
Income-to-needs ratio,		
year prior to birth	.012	−.004
	[.146]	[−.079]
Mother's education		
(HGC by 1984)	−.056	−.065
	[−.865]	[−1.425]
Mother married at child's birth	−.104	.579
	[−.367]	[1.143]
Mother under 18 at child's birth	—	1.562**
		[2.567]
Parental Characteristics		
Mother low birth weight	1.420***	2.637**
	[5.248]	[10.625]
Father low birth weight	2.634***	2.860***
	[10.419]	[10.595]
L^2_{df}	150.28_7	224.35_8
N (groups)	1,255 (395)	3,147 (953)

NOTE: *t*-statistics in brackets.
[a]In the model for African Americans, maternal age is redundant and drops out.
***$p < .001$ **$p < .01$ *$p < .05$

TABLE 2.5. EFFECT OF PARENTAL LOW BIRTH
WEIGHT AND SOCIOECONOMIC CONDITIONS
ON RISK OF FILIAL LOW BIRTH WEIGHT,
GRANDPARENT FIXED-EFFECTS MODELS

Variable	All	Blacks Only	Whites & Others Only
Respondent Characteristics			
Female child	.361	.059	.650*
	[1.934]	[.221]	[2.366]
Firstborn status	.145	.274	.043
	[.812]	[.974]	[.184]
Socioeconomic Variables			
Income-to-needs ratio, year prior to birth	−.014	.109	−.056
	[−.162]	[.146]	[−.513]
Mother's education (HGC by 1984)	−.248**	−.158	−.446**
	[−2.793]	[−1.427]	[−2.814]
Mother married at child's birth	.321	.053	1.090
	[.906]	[.137]	[.972]
Mother under 18 at child's birth	.030	−35.762	.1598
	[.702]	[.000]	[1.416]
Parental Characteristics			
Mother low birth weight	2.035***	1.889**	2.178**
	[4.420]	[2.994]	[2.954]
Father low birth weight	2.378***	1.576**	4.121***
	[5.442]	[3.081]	[3.698]
L^2_{df}	83.14_8	28.63_8	72.19_8
N (groups)	855 (174)	364 (73)	491 (101)
Dropped N (groups)	3,576 (1,174)	920 (322)	2,556 (852)

NOTE: *t*-statistics in brackets.
***$p < .001$ **$p < .01$ *$p < .05$

TABLE 3.1. DESCRIPTIVE STATISTICS
FOR ANALYSES OF LOW BIRTH WEIGHT

African American race	.306
	(.461)
	[—]
Maternal education (highest grade completed [HGC] by 1984)	12.484
	(2.272)
	[—]
Female child	.483
	(.500)
	[.345]
First-born status	.392
	(.488)
	[.395]
Income-to-needs, year prior to birth	2.975
	(2.215)
	[.786]
Mother under 18 years at child's birth	.013
	(.115)
	[.078]
Mother married at child's birth	.904
	(.295)
	[.141]
Mother low birth weight	.073
	(.261)
	[—]
Father low birth weight	.061
	(.240)
	[—]
Filial birth weight (ounces)	119.530
	(20.568)
	[7.845]
N	1,654

NOTE: Respondents born to Panel Study of Income Dynamics (PSID) sample members between 1986 and 1992. Mean values are shown, with standard deviations in parentheses and within-family standard deviations in brackets.

TABLE 3.2. SUBSAMPLE COMPARISONS,
BIRTH WEIGHT ANALYSIS

	Filial Low Birth Weight	Income-to-Needs Ratio Year Prior to Birth	Mother Under 18 at Child's Birth	N
Birth Weight Analysis				
Total sample with LBW information, born ever	.077 [.002]	—	—	14,956
With valid parental information on low birth weight	.067 [.003]	—	—	9,908
Born to sample mothers since 1968	.065 [.003]	—	—	6,004
With complete valid data	.063 [.003]	2.975 [.030]	.013 [.002]	5,596
Only children excluded	.062 [.003]	2.872 [.030]	.012 [.002]	4,975
With discordancy in LBW	.410 [.021]	2.534 [.080]	.015 [.005]	536
Born since 1986 (nonrecalled LBW information)	.051 [.005]	3.666 [.070]	.007 [.002]	1,665

NOTE: Standard deviations in brackets.

TABLE 3.3. EFFECT OF PARENTAL LOW BIRTH WEIGHT AND SOCIOECONOMIC CONDITIONS ON RISK OF FILIAL LOW BIRTH WEIGHT (IN OUNCES), ORDINARY-LEAST-SQUARES REGRESSION MODELS AND SIBLING FIXED-EFFECTS MODELS

	OLS	FE	OLS	With LBW Parent FE	Without LBW Parent FE
Socioeconomic Variables					
Income-to-needs ratio, year prior to birth	.327+ [1.711]	.539 [1.058]	.168 [.887]	8.555** [.887]	.109 [.224]
Mother under 18 at child's birth	-3.982 [-.711]	5.724 [.526]	-3.994 [-.772]	—	5.480 [.538]
Mother married at child's birth	5.031** [2.926]	-3.456 [-.780]	4.640** [2.713]	-16.374 [-1.222]	-3.328** [-.733]
Maternal education (HGC by 1984)	.359 [1.621]	—	.352 [1.603]	—	—
Respondent Characteristics					
Female child	-5.626*** [-5.722]	-3.704* [-2.512]	-5.530*** [-5.658]	18.681** [3.067]	-6.042*** [-5.726]
Firstborn status	-1.424 [-1.489]	-1.685 [-1.239]	-1.302 [-1.367]	3.140 [.612]	-2.182 [-1.626]
African American race	-5.840*** [-4.652]	—	-5.888*** [-4.683]	—	—

Parental Characteristics

	(1)	(2)	(3)	(4)	(5)
Mother low birth weight	-13.828*** [-4.593]	—	-23.179*** [-6.801]	—	—
Father low birth weight	-16.396*** [-5.462]	—	-17.029*** [-3.250]	—	—
Income-Health Interactions					
Mother low birth weight* income-to-needs ratio	—	—	2.894*** [5.598]	—	—
Father low birth weight* Income-to-needs ratio	—	—	.388 [.295]	—	—
Constant	115.886*** [39.386]	123.152*** [26.908]	116.816*** [40.029]	78.638*** [5.179]	127.840*** [27.241]
R^2	.134	.858	.142	.908	.136
N (clusters)	1654 (1216)	1654 (1216)	1654 (1216)	179 (136)	1475 (1080)
Group ID [F-statistic]	—	F(1215,433)*** [1.975]	—	F(135,39)** [2.151]	F(1079,390)*** [1.861]

NOTE: Regression models used with standard errors robust to clustering by mother's ID (t-statistics in brackets).

***$p < .001$ **$p < .01$ *$p < .05$ †$p < .10$

TABLE 4.1. DESCRIPTIVE STATISTICS
FOR ANALYSES OF TIMELY
HIGH SCHOOL GRADUATION

African American race	.331 (.471) [—]
Maternal education (HGC by 1984)	12.111 (2.178) [—]
Female child	.477 (.500) [.343]
Firstborn status	.431 (.495) [.389]
Income-to-needs ratio (birth to age 5)	3.303 (2.153) [.700]
Mother under 18 at child's birth	.035 (.183) [.112]
Mother married at child's birth	.841 (.366) [.160]
Individual low birth weight (1,0)	.067 (.250) [.146]
Individual completes high school by age 19	.445 (.494 females, .402 males) (.497) [.309]
N	1,388

NOTE: Respondents born to PSID sample members between 1986 and 1992.
Mean values shown, with standard deviations in parentheses and within-family
standard deviations in brackets.

TABLE 4.2. SUBSAMPLE COMPARISONS, TIMELY HIGH SCHOOL GRADUATION ANALYSIS

	Individual Low Birth Weight	Income-to-Needs-Ratio (birth to age 5)	Mother under 18 years at Child's Birth	Individual Completes High School by Age 19	N
High School Analysis					
Turned 19 by 1992	.066 [.007]	2.474 [.045]	.037 [.005]	.445 [.013]	1,388
Only children excluded	.063 [.007]	2.420 [.047]	.031 [.005]	.440 [.014]	1,199
With discordancy in HS	.057 [.010]	2.256 [.056]	.029 [.007]	.490 [.021]	581

NOTE: Standard errors in brackets.

TABLE 4.3. EFFECT OF INDIVIDUAL LOW BIRTH WEIGHT
AND MATERNAL SOCIOECONOMIC CONDITIONS ON
PROBABILITY OF TIMELY HIGH SCHOOL GRADUATION,
LOGISTIC REGRESSION MODELS AND SIBLING
FIXED-EFFECTS MODELS

	Logistic Regression	Sibling Fixed Effects	Logistic Regression	Sibling Fixed Effects
Early Life Conditions				
Individual low birth weight	−.555* [−2.386]	−2.195** [−2.833]	−1.446** [−2.696]	−1.331 [−1.038]
Income-to-needs ratio (birth to age 5)	.095* [2.387]	.101 [.774]	.080 [.417]	.112 [.846]
Mother under 18 at child's birth	−.411 [−1.250]	−1.134+ [−1.684]	−.419 [−1.266]	−1.187+ [−1.756]
Mother married at child's birth	.101 [.493]	−.347 [−.729]	.086 [.417]	−.381 [−.790]
Respondent Characteristics				
Female child	.397*** [3.653]	.338+ [1.825]	.391*** [3.568]	.337+ [1.822]
Firstborn status	.232* [2.091]	.011 [.058]	.233* [2.100]	.008 [.044]
African American race	−.005 [−0.036]	—	−.003 [−.019]	—
Maternal education (HGC by 1984)	.022 [.768]	—	.025 [.842]	—
Individual low birth weight* income-to-needs ratio	—	—	.304+ [1.833]	−.518 [−.745]
Constant	−1.094** [−2.777]	—	−1.064** [−2.668]	—
L^2_{df}	40.688	20.566	43.199	21.207
N (clusters)	1,388 (766)	581 (219)	1,388 (766)	581 (219)

NOTE: t-statistics in brackets.
***$p < .001$ **$p < .01$ *$p < .05$ +$p < .10$

TABLE 4.4. EFFECT OF INDIVIDUAL LOW BIRTH WEIGHT AND MATERNAL
SOCIOECONOMIC CONDITIONS ON PROBABILITY ADDITIONAL EDUCATIONAL OUTCOMES,
LOGISTIC REGRESSION MODELS AND SIBLING FIXED-EFFECTS MODELS

	Special Education		Held Back		Disabled	
	Logistic	FE	Logistic	FE	Logistic	FE
Individual low birth weight	.880*	.736	.737*	1.085	1.026*	.537
	(.432)	(.712)	(.350)	(.959)	(.411)	(.652)
Income-to-needs ratio (birth to age 5)	-.019	.956	-.224**	1.010*	-.011	.278
	(.072)	(.536)	(.084)	(.447)	(.070)	(.425)
Mother under 18 at child's birth	.617	35.155	-.056	-34.369	.343	-.918
	(.790)	(.000)	(.590)	(.000)	(.786)	(1.115)
African American race	-.967*	—	-.532*	—	-.825*	—
	(.390)		(.232)		(.374)	
Female child	-.339	-.770	-.769***	-1.471***	-.363	-1.143*
	(.280)	(.520)	(.220)	(.440)	(.279)	(.494)
Firstborn status	-.210	.114	-.017	.111	.233	.427
	(.463)	(.514)	(.221)	(.429)	(.278)	(.584)
Maternal education (HGC by 1984)	-.015	—	-.171***	—	-.024	—
	(.068)		(.052)		(.067)	
Constant	-2.284	—	.236	—	-1.978	—
	(1.060)		(.796)		(1.051)	
Model chi-square$_{(df)}$	11.454(7)	10.42(5)	47.508(7)	24.03(5)	12.108(7)	6.65(5)
N (groups)	1,057 (317)	106 (38)	1,056 (317)	1,52 (54)	1,056 (317)	105 (38)

NOTE: Standard deviations in parentheses.

TABLE 4.5. DESCRIPTIVE STATISTICS FOR
TWIN ANALYSES, BY DISCORDANCY AND SEX

Variable	Total	Discordant	Mixed Sex	Same Sex	Boys Only	Girls Only
Infant death	.029 (.168)	.500 (.500)	.500 (.500)	.500 (.500)	.500 (.500)	.500 (.500)
Neonatal death	.024 (.153)	.321 (.467)	.323 (.468)	.320 (.466)	.316 (.465)	.325 (.468)
Postneonatal death	.005 ($n = 265,503$) (.073)	.264 ($n = 4,479$) (.441)	.261 ($n = 1,335$) (.440)	.265 ($n = 3,144$) (.441)	.269 ($n = 1,745$) (.444)	.259 ($n = 1,399$) (.439)
Firstborn status (of twin pair)	.500 (.500)	.500 (.500)	.500 (.500)	.500 (.500)	.500 (.500)	.500 (.500)
Female child	.498 (.500)	.464 (.499)	.500 (.500)	.448 (.497)	—	—
Individual birth weight	5.24 (1.48)	3.24 (1.76)	3.21 (1.80)	3.25 (1.74)	3.32 (1.83)	3.16 (1.71)
Difference in weight	.633 (.585)	.614 (.700)	.607 (.694)	.617 (.702)	.615 (.720)	.619 (.679)
N	272,004	6,594	1,972	4,622	2,550	2,072

NOTE: Mean values are shown, with standard deviations in parentheses.

TABLE 4.6. EFFECT OF INDIVIDUAL
BIRTH WEIGHT ON INFANT MORTALITY,
BY SEX, TWIN FIXED-EFFECTS MODELS

Variable	Total	Mixed Sex	Same Sex	Boys Only	Girls Only
Firstborn status (of twin pair)	−.056** [−1.54]	−.186** [−2.73]	−.007 [−.15]	−.063 [−1.08]	.063 [.97]
Female child	−.425*** [−6.26]	−.456*** [−6.38]	—	—	—
Individual birth weight	−.748*** [−15.06]	−.892*** [−8.96]	−.703*** [−12.24]	−.688*** [−8.87]	−.720*** [−8.43]
N	6,594	1,972	4,622	2,550	2,072

NOTE: t-statistics in brackets
***$p < .001$ **$p < .01$

TABLE 4.7. EFFECT OF INDIVIDUAL BIRTH
WEIGHT ON NEONATAL INFANT MORTALITY,
BY SEX—TWIN FIXED-EFFECTS MODELS

Variable	Total	Mixed Sex	Same Sex	Boys Only	Girls Only
Firstborn status (of twin pair)	−.032 [−.72]	−.107 [−1.28]	−.010 [−.18]	−.048 [−.67]	.037 [.47]
Female child	−.490*** [−5.90]	−.545*** [−6.15]	—	—	—
Individual birth weight	−.843*** [−13.26]	−1.097*** [−8.01]	−.766*** [−10.67]	−.749*** [−7.76]	−.786*** [−7.32]
N	4,470	1,342	3,128	1,722	1,406

NOTE: t-statistics in brackets.
***$p < .001$

TABLE 4.8. EFFECT OF INDIVIDUAL BIRTH
WEIGHT ON POSTNEONATAL INFANT MORTALITY,
BY SEX—TWIN FIXED-EFFECTS MODELS

Variable	Total	Mixed Sex	Same Sex	Boys Only	Girls Only
Firstborn status (of twin pair)	−.091 [−1.53]	−.269* [−2.42]	−.018 [−.26]	−.082 [−.86]	.108 [.60]
Female child	−.314** [−2.80]	−.305** [−2.64]	—	—	—
Individual birth weight	−.556*** [−7.06]	−.550*** [−3.87]	−.562*** [−5.92]	−.545*** [−4.25]	−.585*** [−4.14]
N	2,364	698	1,666	940	726

NOTE: Conditional on both infants living past thirty days; t-statistics in brackets.
***$p < .001$ **$p < .01$ *$p < .05$

Notes

CHAPTER I

1. Martin, J., Hamilton, B., Ventura, S., Menacher, F., & Park, M. (2002). Births: Final data for 1999. *National Vital Statistics Reports, 50(5)*. Hyattsville, MA: National Center for Health Statistics.

2. Bennett, F. (1997). The LBW, premature infant. In R. Gross, D. Spiker, & C. Haynes (Eds.). *Helping low birth weight, premature babies: The infant health and development program* (pp. 3–16). Stanford, CA: Stanford University Press.

3. Charles, A. (2001, May 15). Scientists find faulty DNA clue to breast cancer. *The Independent*, p. 4; Hensley, S. (2001, May 15). Gene linked to breast cancer yields secrets. *Wall Street Journal*, p. B16; Talan, J. (1998, December 22) Left-handed? Right-handed? Geneticist offers clues. *Newsday*, p. Z06; Gene may affect anxiety disorder. (2001, April 32). *San Diego Union-Tribune*, p. A11; Thomson, A. (2001, July 20). Homosexuality may be in the genes. *The Toronto Star*, p. 4; Maugh, T., & Springer, S. (1997, July 9). In the genes? Doctors may be able to predict if a fighter is susceptible to chronic brain damage. *Los Angeles Times*, p. 1; Gene may predispose some boxers to brain trauma, study finds. (1997, July 9). *Star Tribune*, p. 9A.

4. Breast-fed babies' IQs higher, study says. (1999, September 23). *The Gazette*, p. B1; Benefits of breastfeeding could last for years. (1998, January 9). *The Toronto Star*, p. D2. But some authors have suggested that causation may work in the opposite direction; mothers may be more likely to breast-feed healthier babies in the first place. See Rosenzweig, R., & Wolpin, K. (1988).

Heterogeneity, intra-family distribution and child health. *Journal of Human Resources, 23,* 437–61.

5. Peterson, R. (1997, July 31). Nurturing may play a role in intelligence. *USA Today,* p. 1D.

6. Eskenazi, B., Prehn, A., & Christianson, R. (1995). Passive and active maternal smoking as measured by serum cotinine: The effects on birth weight. *American Journal of Public Health, 85,* 395–98; English, P., Paul, B., Eskenazi, B., & Christianson, R. (1994). Black-white differences in serum cotinine levels among pregnant women and subsequent effects on infant birth weight. *American Journal of Public Health, 84,* 1439–43; Lieberman, E., Gremy, I., & Lang, J. (1994). Low birthweight and the timing of fetal exposure to maternal smoking. *American Journal of Public Health, 94,* 1127–31; Davis, D. (1991). Paternal smoking and fetal health. *Lancet, 337,* 123.

7. Alderman, B., Baron, A., & Salvitz, D. (1987). Maternal exposure to neighborhood carbon monoxide and risk of low infant birth weight. *Public Health Report, 102,* 410–14.

8. Conley, D., Bennett, N., & Li, J. (1999). *Is biology destiny or destiny biology? Poverty, education and intergenerational aspects of low birth weight.* Unpublished manuscript; Aber, J., Bennett, N., Conley, D., & Li, J. (1997). The effects of poverty on child health and development. *Annual Review of Public Health, 18,* 463–83.

9. Aber, J., Bennett, N., Conley, D., & Li, J. (1997); Rogers, I., Emmett, P., Baker, D., & Golding, J. (1998). Financial difficulties, smoking habits, composition of the diet and birth weight in a population of pregnant women in the Southwest of England. *European Journal of Clinical Nutrition, 52(4),* 251–60; Avruch, S., & Cackley, A. (1995). Savings achieved by giving WIC benefits to women prenatally. *Public Health Reports, 110,* 27–34.

10. O'Campo, P., Xue, X., Wang, M., & Caughy, M. (1997). Neighborhood risk factors for low birth weight in Baltimore: A multilevel analysis. *American Journal of Public Health, 80,* 1113–19; Roberts, E. (1997). Neighborhood social environments and the distribution of low birth weight in Chicago. *American Journal of Public Health, 87,* 597–603.

11. Stephan, N., & Gilman, S. (1991). Appropriating the idioms of science: The rejection of scientific racism. In D. LaCapra (Ed.). *The bonds of race: Perspectives on hegemony and resistance* (pp. 72–103). Ithaca: Cornell University Press; Mosse, G. (1981). *Toward the final solution: A history of European racism.* New York: H. Fertig.

12. Herrnstein, R., & Murray, C. (1996). *The bell curve: Intelligence and class struggle in American life.* New York: Free Press.

13. Lewontin, R. (2000). *The triple helix: Gene, organism and environment.* Cambridge, MA: Harvard University Press, p. 5.

14. Jencks, C., Smith, M., Acland, H., Bane, J., Cohen, D., Gintis, H., et al. (1973). *Inequality: A reassessment of the effects of family and schooling in America.* New York: Basic Books.

15. For a discussion of emergent genetics, see Anderson, P. (1972). More is different: Broken symmetry and the nature of the hierarchical structure of science. *Science, 177(4047),* 393–96.

16. Jencks, C., Smith, M., Acland, H., Bane, J., Cohen, D., Gintis, H., et al. (1973), p. 69.

17. See Aber, J., Bennett, N., Conley, D., & Li, J. (1997) for a review of this evidence.

18. Bugental, D., Blue, J., & Jeffrey, L. (1990). Caregiver beliefs and dysphoric affect directed to difficult children. *Developmental Psychology, 26,* 631–38.

19. Jencks, C., Smith, M., Acland, H., Bane, J., Cohen, D., Gintis, H., et al. (1973), pp. 69–71.

20. Wang, X., Zuckerman, B., Coffman, G., & Corwin, M. (1995). Familial aggregation of low birth weight among whites and blacks in the United States. *New England Journal of Medicine, 333,* 1744–49.

21. Miller, J. (1994). Birth order, interpregnancy interval and birth outcomes among Filipino infants. *Journal of Biosocial Science, 26,* 243–59; Conley, D., Bennett, N., & Li, J. (1999); Aber, J., Bennett, N., Conley, D., & Li, J. (1997).

22. Gross, R., Spiker, D., & Haynes, C. (Eds.). (1997). *Helping low birth weight, premature babies: The infant health and development program.* Stanford, CA: Stanford University Press.

23. Smith, T., Young, B., Bae, Y., Choy, S., & Alsalam, N. (1997). *The condition of education* (U.S. Department of Education, National Center for Educational Statistics Report No. 97-388). Washington, DC: U.S. Government Printing Office.

24. National Center for Educational Statistics. (2001, March). *Digest of Educational Statistics.* (Table 248). Washington, DC: Author; See also: Hacker, A. (2001, April 11). How are women doing? *New York Review of Books, 49(6),* 63–66.

25. Himmelmann, A., Svensson, A., & Handsson, L. (1994). Relation of maternal blood pressure during pregnancy to birth weight and blood pressure in children: The Hypertension Study. *Journal of Internal Medicine, 235,* 347–52; Avruch, S., & Cackley, A. (1995); Rogers, I., Emmett, P., Baker, D., & Golding, J. (1998).

26. Gross, R., Spiker, D., & Haynes, C. (Eds.). (1997).

27. Conley, D., Bennett, N., & Li, J. (1999); Aber, J., Bennett, N., Conley, D., & Li, J. (1997).

28. Aber, J., Bennett, N., Conley, D., & Li, J. (1997); Gross, R., Spiker, D., & Haynes, C. (Eds.). (1997).

29. Wang, W., Zuckerman, B., Coffman, G., & Corwin, M. (1995).

30. Corner, B. (1960). *Prematurity: The diagnosis, care and disorders of the premature infant.* Springfield, IL: Thomas Books.

31. Sepkowitz, S. (1995). International ranking of infant mortality and the U.S.: Vital Statistics natality data collecting system—failures and success. *International Journal of Epidemiology, 24,* 583–88.

32. Sepkowitz, S. (1995).

33. Sachs, B., Fretts, R., Gardner, R., Hellersien, S., Wampler, N., & Wise, P. (1995). The impact of extreme prematurity and congenital abnormalities on the interpretation of international comparisons of infant mortality. *Obstetrics and Gynecology, 85,* 941–46.

34. Reed, D., & Stanley, F. (Eds.). (1977). *The epidemiology of prematurity*. Baltimore, MD: Urban and Schwarzenberg; Kramer, M., Platt, R., Yang, H., McNamara, H., & Usher, R. (1999). Are all growth-restricted newborns created equal(ly)? *Pediatrics, 103,* 599–602; Kallan, J. (1993). Race, intervening variables, and two components of low birth weight. *Demography, 30,* 489–506.

35. Frisbie, W., Forbes, D., & Pullman, S. (1996). Compromised birth outcomes and infant mortality among racial and ethnic groups. *Demography, 33,* 469–81.

36. Bennett, F. (1997).

37. Luke, B., Williams, L., Minogue, J., & Keith, L. (1993). The changing pattern of infant morality in the United States: The role of prenatal factors and their obstetrical implications. *International Journal of Gynecology and Obstetrics, 40,* 199–212.

38. Centers for Disease Control, National Center for Health Statistics. (1998). Tables from the Linked Birth/Infant Death File. Retrieved May 16, 2000, from http://www.cdc.gov/nchswww/datawh/statab/unpubd/mortabs.htm

39. Centers for Disease Control, National Center for Health Statistics. (1998).

40. Bennett, F. (1998). Neurodevelopmental outcomes in low birth weight infants: The role of developmental intervention. In R. Guthrie (Ed.). *Neonatal intensive care: Clinics in critical care medicine* (pp. 121–250). New York: Church Livingstone.

41. Partin, M., & Pallonu, A. (1995). Accounting for the recent increase in low birth weight among African Americans. *Focus, 16,* 33–37.

42. Luke, B., Williams, C., Minogue, J., & Keith, L. (1993).

43. Kallan, J. (1993); Collins, J., & David, R. (1993). Race and birth weight in biracial infants. *American Journal of Public Health, 83,* 1125–29; Gould, J., & LeRoy, S. (1998). Socioeconomic status and low birth weight: A racial comparison. *Pediatrics, 82,* 896–904; Geronimus, A. (1996); Hummer, R. (1993). Racial differences in infant mortality in the U.S.: An examination of social and health determinants. *Social Forces, 72,* 529–54.

44. Gould, J., Davey, B., & LeRoy, S. (1989). Socioeconomic differentials and neonatal mortality: Racial comparison of California singletons. *Pediatrics, 83,* 181–86.

45. Starfield, B., Shapiro, S., Weiss, J., Liang, K., Ra, K., Paige, D., et al. (1991). Race, family income, and low birth weight. *American Journal of Epidemiology, 134,* 1167–74.

46. Collins, J., & Shay, K. (1994). Prevalence of low birth weight among Hispanic infants with United States–born and foreign-born mothers: The effect of urban poverty. *American Journal of Epidemiology, 139,* 184–92.

47. Duncan, G., & Laren, D. (1990, February 13). *Neighborhood and family correlates of low birth weight: Preliminary results on births to black women from the PSID-geocode file* (Research report). Ann Arbor, MI: University of Michigan, Survey Research Center.

48. See, for instance, Bakketeig, L., Jacobsen, G., Hoffman, H., Lindmark, G., Bergsjo, P., et al. (1993). Pre-pregnancy risk factors of small-for-gestational age births among parous women in Scandinavia. *Acta Obstetrica Gynecologica*

Scandinavia, 72, 273–79; Lang, J., Lieberman, E., & Cohen, A. (1996). A comparison of risk factors for preterm labor and term small-for-gestational age birth. *Epidemiology, 7,* 369–76; Overspect, M., & Moss, A. (1991). *Children's exposure to environmental cigarette smoke before and after birth* (Advanced Data Report No. 202). Hyattsville, MA: National Center for Health Statistics.

49. Sulloway, F. (1996).

50. Pearl, R., & Donahue, M. (1995). Four years after a pre-term birth: Children's development and their mother's beliefs and expectations. *Journal of Pediatric Psychology, 20,* 363–70; Adairs, L., & Popkin, B. (1996). Low birth weight reduces the likelihood of breast-feeding among Filipino infants. *Journal of Nutrition, 126,* 103–12.

51. Corner, B. (1960).

52. Dunn, H., Crichton, R., Grunau, A., McBurney, A., McCormmick, A., Roberston, A., et al. (1980). Neurological, psychological and educational sequelae of low birth weight. *Brain Development, 2,* 57–67.

53. Breslow, N., PelDotto, J., Brown, G., Kumar, S., Ezhuthachan, K., Hunfnagle, K., et al. (1994). A gradient relationship between low birth weight and IQ at age 6 years. *Archives of Pediatric and Adolescent Medicine, 148,* 377–83; Brooks-Gunn, J., Klebanov, P., & Duncan, G. (1996). Ethnic differences in children's intelligence test scores: Role of economic deprivation, home environment and maternal characteristics. *Child Development, 67,* 396–408.

54. Dobson, B. (1994). A WIC primer. *Journal of Human Lactation, 10,* 199–202.

55. Michaelis, R., Asenbauer, C., Buchwald-Senal, M., Haas, G., & Krageboh-Mann, I. (1993). Transitory neurological findings in a population of at risk infants. *Early Human Development, 34,* 143–53; Roberston, C., Hrynchyshyn, G., Etches, P., & Pain, K. (1992). Population-based study of the incidence, complexity and severity of neurological disability among survivors weighing 500 through 1250 grams at birth: A comparison of two birth cohorts. *Pediatrics, 990,* 750–55.

56. McCormick, M., Stemmler, M., Bernbaum, J., & Farran, A. (1986). The very low birth weight transport goes home: Impact on the family. *Journal of Developmental Behavioral Pediatrics, 10,* 86–91.

57. Gertz, L., Dobson, V., & Luna, B. (1994). Development of grating acuity, letter acuity and visual fields in small-for-gestational-age preterm infants. *Early Human Development, 40,* 59–71; Aber, J., Bennett, N., Conley, D., & Li, J. (1997); Scott, D., & Spiker, D. (1989). Research on the sequelae of prematurity: Early learning, early interventions and later outcomes. *Seminal perinatology, 13,* 495–505; Friedman, S., Jacobs, B., & Weithmann, M. (1982). Preterms of low medical risk: Spontaneous behaviors and soothability at expected date of birth. *Infant behavioral development, 5,* 3–10.

58. Bennett, F. (1997).

59. McCormick, M., Shapiro, S., & Starfield, B. (1980). Rehospitalization in the first years of life for high-risk survivors. *Pediatrics, 66,* 991–99; Tekolste, K., & Bennett, F. (1987). The high risk infant: Transitions in health, development and family during the first years of life. *Journal of Perinatology, 7,* 368–77.

60. Bader, D., Kamos, A., Lwe, C., Platzker, A., Stabile, M., & Keens, T. (1987). Childhood sequelae of infant lung disease: Exercise and pulmonary function abnormalities after bronchoulmonary dysplasia. *Journal of Pediatrics, 110,* 693–99.

61. McCormick, M., Stemmler, M., Bernbaum, J., & Farran, A. (1986).

62. Bennett, F. (1997).

63. Sorensen, H., Sabroe, S., Olsen, J., Rothman, K., Gillman, M., & Fischer, P. (1997). Birth weight and cognitive function in young adult life: Historical cohort study. *British Medical Journal, 315,* 401–3.

64. Hack, M., Flannery, D., Schluchter, M., Cartar, L., Borawski, E., & Klein, N. (2002). Outcomes in young adulthood for very low birth weight infants. *The New England Journal of Medicine, 346,* 149–57.

65. Bradley, R., Whiteside, L., Mundform, D., Casey, P., Kehheher, K., & Pope, S. (1994). Early indications of resilience and their relation to experiences in the home environments of low birth weight, premature children living in poverty. *Child Development, 65,* 346–60.

66. See, for instance, Aber, J., Bennett, N., Conley, D., & Li, J. (1997).

67. Wang, X., Zuckerman, G., Coffman, G., & Corwin, M. (1995).

68. Personal communication at Robert Wood Johnson Foundation's Clinical Scholar's Meeting. (1997).

69. Amante, A., Borgiani, P., Gimelfarb, A., & Gloria-Bottini, F. (1996). Interethnic variability in birth weight and genetic background: A study of placental alkaline phosphates. *American Journal of Physical Anthropology, 1010,* 449–53.

70. Behrman, J., & Rosenzweig, M. (2001). *The returns to increasing body weight.* (Working Paper No. 01-052). Philadelphia, PA: University of Pennsylvania, Pennsylvania Institute for Economic Research.

71. Brooks, A., Johnson, P., Pawson, M., & Abdalla, H. (1995). Birth weight: Nature or nurture? *Early Human Development, 42,* 29–35.

72. Copley, J. (1999). A runt for life. *New Scientist, 161,* 14.

73. See, for a summary, Duncan, G., & Brooks-Gunn, J. (1997). Income effects across the life span: Integration and interpretation. In G. Duncan & J. Brooks-Gunn (Eds.). *Consequences of growing up poor* (pp. 596–610). New York: Russell Sage Foundation.

74. Martinez, F., Wright, A., Taussig, L., & the Group Health Medical Associates. (1994). The effect of paternal smoking on the birthweight of newborns whose mothers did not smoke. *American Journal of Public Health, 89,* 1489–91.

75. Daniels, C. (1997). Between fathers and fetuses: The social construction of male reproduction and the politics of fetal harm. *Signs, 22,* 579–616.

76. Freidler, H., & Wheeling, H. (1997). Behavioral effects in offspring of male mice injected with opioids prior to mating. In *Protracted effects of perinatal drug dependence, vol. 2. Pharmacology, Biochemistry and Behavior* (pp. s23–s28). Fayetteville, NY: ANKHO International.

77. Colie, C. (1993). Male mediated teratogenesis. *Reproductive Toxicology, 7,* 3–9.

78. Stellman, S., & Stellman, J. (1980).

79. Averett, S., & Korenman, S. (1996). The economic reality of the beauty myth. *Journal of Human Resources, 31*, 304–30; Pagan, J., & Davila, A. (1997). Obesity, occupational attainment and earnings. *Social Science Quarterly, 78*, 756–70.

80. Averett, S., & Korenman, S. (1996); Rissahen, A. (1996). The economic and psychological consequences of obesity. *Origins and Consequences of Obesity, 201*, 194–96; Roehling, M. (1999). Weight-based discrimination in employment: Psychological and legal aspects. *Personnel Psychology, 52*, 969–1016; Seidell, J. (1998). Societal and personal costs of obesity. *Experimental and Clinical Endocrinology and Diabetes, 106(2)(suppl)*, 7–9.

81. Power, C., & Parsons, T. (2000). Nutritional and other influences in childhood as predictors of adult obesity. *Proceedings of the nutrition society, 59*, 257–72; Sobal, J., & Stunkard, A. (1989). Socioeconomic status and obesity: A review of the literature. *Psychological Bulletin, 105*, 260–75; Stunkard, A. (1996). Socioeconomic status and obesity. *Origins and Consequences of Obesity, 201*, 174–87.

82. Avarette, S., & Korenman, S. (1996).

83. Behrman, J., & Rosenzweig, M. (2001).

84. Berhman, J., & Rosenzweig, M. (2001).

85. Riese, M. (1995). Neonatal temperament in full-term twin pairs discordant for birth weight. *Journal of Development and Behavioral Pediatrics, 15*, 342–47; Riese, M. (1996). Temperamental development to 30 months of age in discordant twin pairs. *Acta geneticae medicae et gemellologiae, 45*, 439–47.

86. Himmelmann, A., Svensson, A., & Handsson, L. (1994); Avruch, S., & Cackley, A. (1995); Rogers, I., Emmett, P., Baker, D., & Golding, J. (1998).

87. Pearl, R., & Donahue, M. (1995); Adairs, L., & Popkin, N. (1996); McCormick, M., Brooks-Gunn, J., Workman-Daniels, K., & Peckham, G. (1993). Maternal rating of child health at school age: Does the Vulnerable Child Syndrome persist? *Pediatrics, 92*, 380–88.

88. Festinger, L. (1957). *A theory of cognitive dissonance.* Stanford: Stanford University Press.

89. Sanderson, M., Williams, M., White, E., Daling, J., Holt, K., Malone, K., et al. (1998). Validity and reliability of subject and mother reporting of perinatal factors. *American Journal of Epidemiology, 147*, 136–40.; Lederman, S., & Paxton, A. (1998). Maternal reporting of prepregnancy weight and birth outcome: Consistency and completeness compared with the clinical record. *Maternal and Child Health Journal, 2*, 123–26.

CHAPTER 2

1. Hoyert, D., Arias, E., Smith, B., Murphy, S., & Kochanek, K. (2001). Deaths: Final data for 1999. *National Vital Statistics Reports, 49(8)*. Hyattsville, MA: National Center for Health Statistics.

2. Hoyert, D., Arias, E., Smith, B., Murphy, S., & Kochanek, K. (2001).

3. Martin, J., Hamilton, B., Ventura, S., Menacher, F., & Park, M. (2002).

4. Murphy, S. (2000).

5. Hoyert, D., Arias, E., Smith, B., Murphy, S., & Kochanek, K. (2001).

6. Centers for Disease Control, National Center for Health Statistics. (1993). Health, United States, 1992. Hyattsville, MD: Author.

7. Murphy, S. (2000).

8. For a review of these issues see: Williams, D., & Collins, C. (1995).

9. Kreiger, N. (1990). Racial and gender discrimination: Risk factors for high blood pressure? *Social Science and Medicine, 30,* 1273–81; Williams, D. (1994). The concept of race in health services research, 1966–1990. *Health Services Research, 29,* 261–74; Williams, D. (1992). Black-white differences in blood pressure: The role of social factors. *Ethnicity and Disease, 2,* 126–41.

10. Dressler, W. (1993). Health in the African American community: Accounting for health inequalities. *Medical Anthropology Quarterly, 7,* 320–45.

11. Schachter, J., Lachin, J., & Wimberly, F. (1976). Newborn heart rate and blood pressure: Relation to race and socioeconomic class. *Psychosomatic Medicine, 38,* 390–98.

12. Columbia University, National Center for Children in Poverty (2001, June). Child poverty fact sheet: June 2001. Retrieved September 21, 2002, from http://cpmcnet.columbia.edu/dept/nccp/ycpf-01.html

13. Ventura, S., Martin, J., Curtin, S., Mathews, T., & Park, M. (2000).

14. Maxwell, N. (1994). The effects of black-white wage differences in the quality and quantity of education. *Industrial Labor Relations and Review, 47,* 249–64.

15. Bureau of Labor Statistitcs. (2002). Table 10: Employed persons by occupation, race, and sex. Retrieved February 7, 2002, from www.bls.gov/cps

16. Wilson, W. (1978). *The declining significance of race and changing American institutions.* Chicago: University of Chicago Press, 1.

17. Conley, D. (1999).

18. DeBarros, S., & Bennett, C. (1998); Williams, D., & Collins, C. (1995); Conley, D. (1999).

19. West, C. (1993). *Race matters.* Boston: Beacon Press.

20. For a review of this literature, see Williams, D., & Collins, C. (1995).

21. Lieberman, E., Ryan, K., Monson, R., & Schoenbaum, S. (1987). Risk factors accounting for racial differences in premature births. *New England Journal of Medicine, 317,* 743–48.

22. Moss, N., & Carver, K. (1998). The effect of WIC and Medicaid on infant mortality in the United States. *American Journal of Public Health, 88,* 1354–61.

23. Gould, J., & LeRoy, S. (1988); Collins, J., & David, R. (1990).

24. Shmueli, A., & Cullen, M. (2000). Birth weight, maternal age, and education: New observations from Connecticut and Virginia. *Yale Journal of Biological Medicine, 72,* 245–58.

25. Wolff, E. (2000). Recent trends in wealth ownership, 1983–1998. The Jerome Levy Institute Working Paper no. 300.

26. Conley, D. (1999).

27. Mare, R. (1990). Socioeconomic careers and differential morality among older men in the U.S. In J. Vallin, S. D'Souza, & A. Palloni (Eds.), *Measure-*

ment and analysis of mortality—New approaches. (pp. 362–87). Oxford, UK: Clarendon.

28. Goldblatt, P. (1990) *Longitudinal study: Mortality and social organization.* London: Her Majesty's Stationery Office.

29. Catalano, R. (1991). The health effects of economic insecurity. *American Journal of Public Health, 81,* 1148–58; Catalano, R., & Sexner, S. (1992). The effect of ambient threats to employment on low birth weight. *Journal of Health and Social Behavior, 33,* 363–77.

30. For a discussion of wealth inheritance, see Chiteji, N., & Stafford, F. (2000). Asset ownership across generations. The Levy Institute for Economics Working Paper no. 314. For more general estimates, see Kotlikoff, L., & Summers, L. (1981). The role of intergenerational transfers in aggregate capital accumulation. *Journal of Political Economy, 89,* 706–32; Modigliani, F. (1988). The role of intergenerational transfers and life cycle saving in the accumulation of wealth. *Journal of Economic Perspectives, 2,* 15–40.

31. U.S. Census Bureau. (2000). American housing survey of the United States, 1999: Table 2-1. Introductory characteristics—occupied units. Retrieved January 2002 from www.census.gov/hhes/www/housing/ahs/ahs99/ahs99.htm

32. Potter, L. (1991). Socioeconomic determinants of white and black males' life expectancy differentials, 1980. *Demography, 28,* 303–21; Polednak, A. (1997). *Segregation, poverty and mortality in urban African Americans.* Oxford: Oxford University Press; Polednak, A. (1991). Black-white differentials in infant mortality in 38 standard metropolitan statistical areas. *American Journal of Public Health, 81,* 1480–82; LeClere, F., Richard, R., & Peters, K. (1997). Ethnicity and mortality in the United States: Individual and neighborhood level correlates. *Social Forces, 76,* 169–98; LaVeist, T. (1992). The political empowerment and health status of African Americans: Mapping a new territory. *American Journal of Sociology, 97,* 1080–95; LaVeist, T. (1993). Segregation, poverty and empowerment: Health consequences for African Americans. *Milbank Quarterly, 71,* 41–64.

33. For a review, see Ellen, I. (2000). Is segregation bad for your health? The case of low birth weight. Brookings-Wharton Papers on Urban Affairs; Polednak, A. (1991).

34. Ellen, I. (2000) The precise degree of decline depends on the measurement of segregation used.

35. Troutt, D. (1993). The thin red line: How the poor still pay more. San Francisco Consumers Union of the United States, West Coast Regional Office.

36. Rosenbaum, E. (1997). Racial/ethnic differences in home ownership and housing quality. *Social Problems, 43,* 403–26.

37. Ellen, I. (2000). Again, the degree of decline depends on the measurement of segregation.

38. For a discussion of the Black report, see Vagero, D., & Illsley, R. (1995). Explaining health inequality: Beyond Black and Barker. *European Sociological Review, 11,* 219–41.

39. Pattillo-McCoy, M., & Heflin, C. (1999). Poverty in the family: Siblings of the black and white middle classes. Paper presented at the Annual Meeting of the American Sociological Association, Chicago, IL.

40. Hummer, R. (1996). Black-white differences in health and mortality: A review and conceptual model. *Sociological Quarterly, 37,* 108.

41. Dressler, W. (1993).

42. Dressler, W. (1993); Klag, M., Whelton, D., Coresh, J., Grim, C., & Kuller, L. (1991). The association of skin color with blood pressure in U.S. blacks with low socioeconomic status. *Journal of the American Medical Association, 265,* 599–602.

43. Kreiger, N. (1990); Williams, D., Lavizzo-Maourey, R., & Warren, R. (1994). The concept of race and health status in America. *Public Health Reports, 109,* 26–42.

44. James, S. (1994). John Henryism and the health of African Americans. *Culture, Medicine and Psychiatry, 18,* 163–82.

45. For a discussion, see James, S. (1994); Last, J. (Ed.). (1986). *Hypertension in Public Health and Preventative Medicine* (12th ed.). Norwalk, CT: Appelton-Century-Crofts.

46. See, for a discussion, James, S. (1994).

47. James, S. (1994), 1167.

48. Geronimus, A. (1996).

49. Mcknight, J. (1985). Health and empowerment. *Canadian Journal of Public Health, 76(suppl),* S37–S38

50. LaVeist, T. (1992).

51. Morenoff, J. (2001). *Place, race, and health: Neighborhood sources of group disparities in birthweight* (PSC Research Report No. 01-482). Ann Arbor: University of Michigan, Population Studies Center.

52. For discussions of these trends see: Guendelman, S., Gould, J., Hudes, M., & Eskenazi, B. (1990). Generational differences in perinatal health among the Mexican American population: Findings from HANES. *American Journal of Public Health, 80,* 61–65; Schribner, R., & Dwyer, J. (1989). Acculturation and low birthweight among Latinos in the Hispanic HANES. *American Journal of Public Health, 79,* 1263–67; Cervantes, A., Keith, L., & Wyshak, G. (1999). Adverse birth outcomes among native-born and immigrant women: Replicating national evidence regarding Mexicans at the local level. *Maternal and Child Health Journal, 3,* 99–109.

53. Scribner, R., & Dwyer, J. (1989).

54. David, R., & Collins, J. (1997). Differing birth weight among infants of U.S.-born blacks, African-born blacks and U.S.-born whites. *New England Journal of Medicine, 337,* 1209–14; Pallotto, E., Collins, J., & David, R. (2000). Enigma of maternal race and infant birth weight: A population-based study of U.S.-born black and Caribbean-born black women." *American Journal of Epidemiology, 151,* 1080–85.

55. Borjas, G. (1990). Immigration and self selection. In R. Freeman & R. Aboard (Eds.), *Immigration, Trade and the Labor Market.* (pp. 29–76). Chicago, IL: University of Chicago Press; Massey, D. (1993). Latinos, poverty and the underclass: A new agenda for research. *Hispanic Journal of Behavioral Sciences, 15,* 449–75.

56. Landale, N., Oropesa, R., & Golman, B. (2000).

57. Landale, N., Oropesa, R., & Gorman, B. (2000).

58. Frisbie, W., Cho, Y., & Hummer, R. (2001). Immigration and the health of Asian and American Pacific Islander adults in the U.S. *American Journal of Epidemiology, 153,* 372–80.

59. Frisbie, W., Forbes, D., & Pullman, S. (1996).

60. Kramer, M., Platt, R., Yang, H., McNamara, H., & Usher, R. (1999); Kallan, J. (1993).

61. Kallan, J. (1993).

62. Kallan, J. (1993).

63. Goodman, R., & Moltusky, A. (1984); Nash, K., & Kramer, K. (1993).

64. Stevens, J. (in press). Symbolic matter: DNA and other linguistic stuff. *Social Text.*

65. Alexander, G., Tompkins, M., Altekruse, J., & Hornung, C. (1985). Racial differences in the relation of birth weight and gestational age to neonatal mortality. *Public Health Reports, 100(5),* 539–47.

66. For a summary of these studies see: Mangold, W., & Powell-Griner, E. (1991). Race of parents and infant birthweight in the United States. *Social Biology, 38,* 13–27.

67. Mangold, W., & Powell-Griner, E. (1991).

68. Parker, J., & Schoendorf, K. (1992).

69. Elwood, C., & Hoem, J. (1999). Low-weight neonatal survival paradox in the Czech Republic. *American Journal of Epidemiology, 149,* 447–53.

70. David, R., & Collins, J. (1997).

71. For a review, see Hummer, R. (1996); Foster, H. (1997). The enigma of low birth weight and race. *New England Journal of Medicine, 337,* 1232–33.

72. Cooper, R. (1994). A note on the biological concept of race and its application in epidemiology research. *American Heart Journal, 108,* 715–23.

73. Stevens, J. (in press).

74. Duster, T. (1990). *Back door to eugenics.* New York: Routledge.

75. Duster, T. (1990), 51–52.

76. Murphy, S. (2000).

77. DES Action. Health risks and care for DES daughters. Retrieved January 12, 2002, from http://www.desaction.org; National Institute of Environmental Health Services, National Toxicology Program. (n.d.). Known carcinogen: diethylstilbestrol (CAS No. 56-53-1). Research Triangle Park, NC: Author. Retrieved January 12, 2002, from http://ntpserver.niehs.nih.gov/htdocs/ARC /ARC_KC/Diethylstilbestrol.html; Centers for Disease Control, National Center for Environmental Health. (n.d.). CDC's lead poisoning prevention program. Retrieved January 12, 2002, from http://www.cdc.gov/nceh/lead/lead .htm; Centers for Disease Control, National Center for Environmental Health. (2001, December 22). Blood lead levels in young children: United States and selected states, 1996–1999. *Morbidity and Mortality Weekly Report, 49(50),* 1133–37. Retrieved January 12, 2002, from http://www.cdc.gov/mmwr/preview /mmwrhtml/mm4950a3.htm

78. Centers for Disease Control, National Center for Environmental Health. (n.d.).; Centers for Disease Control, National Center for Environmental Health. (2001, December 22).

79. Thanks to Elizabeth Wrigley-Field for this suggestion.

CHAPTER 3

1. We are speaking here of industrialized countries. Nonindustrialized countries have not experienced the same epidemiological shifts, and thus infectious diseases, rarely seen in industrialized countries, are still quite prevalent in many nonindustrialized nations. Nonindustrialized countries have not benefited from the technological innovations or increases in standards of living that have extended life expectancies in industrialized countries and ultimately led to shifts in disease patterns.

For a recent discussion of inequalities in global public health see: Epstein, H. (2001, April 12). Time of indifference. *New York Review of Books, 48(3),* 12–15. For a discussion of epidemiological shifts in industrialized countries see: Link, B. (1995). Social conditions as fundamental causes of disease. *Journal of Health and Social Behavior (Extra issue),* 80–94; McKinlay, J., & McKinlay, S. (1997). Medical measures and the decline of mortality. In P. Conrad (Ed.), *The sociology of health and illness,* 5th ed. (pp. 10–23). New York: St. Martin's Press.

2. Villermé, L. (1840). *Tableau d'etat physique et moral des ouvriers, Vol.* 2. Paris: Renouard.

3. Davey-Smith, G., Shipley, M., & Rose, G. (1990). Magnitude and causes of socioeconomic differentials in mortality: Further evidence from the Whitehall study. *Journal of Epidemiology and Community Health, 44,* 265–70.

4. Engles, F. (1967). *The process of capitalist production* (S. Moore & E. Aveling, Eds. & Trans.). New York: International Publishers. (Original work published 1867)

5. Gould, J., Davey, B., & LeRoy, S. (1989).

6. Mackenback, J. (1992). Socio-economic health differences in the Netherlands: A review of recent empirical findings. *Social Science and Medicine, 34,* 213–26.

7. Illsley, R., & Mulley, K. (1985). The health needs of disadvantaged client groups. In W. Holland, R. Detels, & G. Knox (Eds.). *Oxford textbook of public health* (pp. 389–402). Oxford, UK: Oxford University Press; Williams, D., & Collins, C. (1995).

8. Evans, R., Barer, M., & Marmot, T. (Eds.). (1994). *Why are some people healthy and others are not? Determinants of health of populations.* New York: DeGruyter Press; Adler, N., Boyce, T., & Chesney, M. (1994). SES and health: The challenge of the gradient. *American Psychologist, 49,* 15–24.

9. Sapolsky, R. (1994). *Why zebras don't get ulcers: A guide to stress, stress related diseases and coping.* New York: W. H. Freeman; Sapolsky, R. (1993). Endrocrinology alfresco: Psycho-endocrine studies of wild baboons. *Recent Progress in Hormone Research, 48,* 437–68; Cassel, J. (1976). The contribution of the social environment to host resistance. *American Journal of Epidemiology, 104,* 107–23.

10. Link, B., Northridge, M., Phelan, J., & Ganz, M. (1998). Social epidemiology and the fundamental causes concept: On the structuring of effective cancer screens by socioeconomic status. *Milbank Quarterly, 76,* 375–402;

Link, B., & Phelan, J. (1995). Social conditions as fundamental causes of disease. *Journal of Health and Social Behavior (extra issue)*, 80–94.

11. Link, B., Northridge, M., Phelan, J., & Ganz, M. (1998).

12. Pappas, G., Queen, S., Hadden, W., & Fisher, G. (1993). The increasing disparity between socioeconomic groups in the Untied States, 1960 to 1986. *New England Journal of Medicine, 329*, 103–15; Kitagawa, E., & Hauser, P. (1973). *Differential mortality in the United States: A study in socioeconomic epidemiology*. Cambridge, MA: Harvard University Press.

13. House, J., Kessler, R., Herzog, A., Mero, R., Kinner, A., & Breslow, M. (1990). Age, socioeconomic status and health. *Milbank Quarterly, 68*, 383–411.

14. Marmot, M., Smith, G., Stansgeld, S., Patek, C., North, F., Head, J., et al. (1991). Health inequalities among British civil servants: The Whitehall study. *Lancet, 337*, 1387–93; Davey-Smith, G., Shipley, M., & Rose, G. (1990).

15. Smith, C. (1947). The effects of wartime starvation on pregnancy and its products. *American Journal of Obstetric Gynecology, 53*, 599–608; Lumey, L., & Van Poppel, F. (1994). The Dutch Famine of 1944–1945: Mortality and morbidity in past and present generations. *Social Historical Medicine, 7*, 229–46; Stein, Z., Susser, M., Saegner, G., & Marrolla, F. (1975). *Famine and human development: The Dutch hunger winter of 1944–1945*. New York: Oxford University Press.

16. Gortmaker, S. (1979). Poverty and infant mortality in the United States. *American Sociological Review, 44*, 280–97.

17. LaVeist, T. (1990, Winter). Simulating the effects of poverty on the race disparity in post-neonatal mortality. *Journal of Public Health Policy*, 462–73; Starfield, B., Shapiro, S., Wiess, J., Liang, K., Ra, K., Paige, D., et al. (1991).

18. Collins, J., & Shay, K. (1994).

19. For a more thorough discussion of the poverty measure and infant health, see Aber, J., Bennett, N., Conley, D., & Li, J. (1997).

20. Committee on National Statistics, Panel on Poverty and Family Assistance. (1995). *Measuring poverty: A new approach. A report from the NAS panel on poverty and family assistance: Concepts, information needs, and measurement methods*. Washington, DC: Author.

21. Joint Economic Committee. (1989). Washington, DC: U.S. Government Printing Office. For additional discussion, see Aber, J., Bennett, N., Conley, D., & Li, J. (1997).

22. Stevens, R., & Stevens, R. (1974). *Welfare medicine in America: A case study of Medicaid*. New York: The Free Press; Ku, L., Ullman, F., & Almeida, R. (1999). *What counts? Determining Medicaid and CHIP eligibility for children*. (Urban Institute Discussion Paper No. 99-05). Washington, DC: Urban Institute Press.

23. Available at ferret.bls.census.gov/macro/032002/pov/new02_001.htm and www.census.gov/hhes/poverty/threshld/thresho1.html

24. Duncan, G., & Rodgers, W. (1988). Has children's poverty become more persistent? *American Sociological Review, 56*, 361–75.

25. For a discussion of poverty and children's outcomes, see Aber, J., Bennett, N., Conley, D., & Li, J. (1997); Duncan, G., & Brooks-Gunn, J. (Eds.).

(1997). *Consequences of growing up poor.* New York: Russell Sage Foundation; Smith, S., & Dixon, R. (1995). Literacy concepts of low- and middle-class four year olds entering preschool. *Journal of Educational Research, 88,* 243–53; Duncan, G., Brooks-Gunn, J., Yeung, J., & Smith, J. (1998). How much does childhood poverty affect the life chances of children? *American Sociological Review, 63,* 406–23.

26. Smith, C. (1947); Antonov, A. (1947). Children born during the siege of Leningrad in 1947. *Journal of Pediatrics, 30,* 250.

27. Lumey, L., & Stein, A. (1997). In-utero exposure to famine and subsequent fertility: The Dutch famine birth cohort study. *American Journal of Public Health, 87,* 1962–66.

28. Widga, A., & Lewis, N. (1999). Defined, in-home prenatal nutrition intervention for low-income women. *Journal of the American Dietetic Association, 99(9),* 1058–62; Rogers, I., Emmett, P., Baker, D., & Golding, J. (1998).

29. Avruch, S., & Cackley, A. (1995).

30. Roberts, E. (1997).

31. Vaughan, V., & Mkay, J. (1975). *Textbook of pediatrics.* Philadelphia: Saunders; Department of Health and Social Security. (1970). *Confidential inquiry into post-neonatal deaths, 1964–1966* (Reports on Public Medical Subjects No. 125). London: Her Majesty's Stationery Office.

32. Gortmaker, S. (1979).

33. Showstack, J., Budetti, P., & Minkler, D. (1984). Factors associated with birth weight: An exploration of the roles of prenatal care and length of gestation. *American Journal of Public Health, 74,* 1003–8.

34. For a discussion of these different effects, see Collins, J., & David, R. (1992). Differences in neonatal mortality by race, income and prenatal care. *Ethnicity and Disease, 2,* 18–26.

35. Collins, J., & David, R. (1992).

36. Troutt, D. (1993).

37. Lynge, E. (1984). Socioeconomic and occupational morality differentials in Europe. *Sozial-un Praventivmedizin, 29,* 265–67; LeClerc, A., Lert, F., & Goldberg, M. (1984). Les inegalites sociales devant la mort en Grande Bretagne et en France. *Social Science and Medicine, 19,* 479–87; Koskenvuo, M., Kaprio, J., Kesaniemi, A., & Sarna, S. (1978). Differences in mortality from ischemic heart disease by marital status and social class. *Journal of Chronic Disease, 33,* 95–106; Kagamimori, S., Iibuchi, Y., & Fox, A. (1983). A comparison of socioeconomic differences in mortality between Japan, England, and Wales. *World Health Statistics Quarterly, 36,* 119–28; Kaplan, G. (1985). Twenty years of health in Alameda County: The Human Population Laboratory Analysis. Paper presented at the annual meeting of Society for Prospective Medicine, San Francisco.

38. Illsley, R. (1955). Social class selection and class differences in relation to still-births and infant death. *British Medical Journal, 2,* 1520–24.

39. Evans, R., Barer, M., & Marmor, T. (Eds.). (1994).

40. Wilkinson, R. (1986). Income inequality. In R. Wilkinson (Ed.), *Class and health: Research and longitudinal data* (pp. 1–20). London: Tavistock.

41. Wilkinson, R. (1992). Income distribution and life expectancy. *British Medical Journal, 304,* 165–68.

42. Kennedy, B., Kawachi, I., & Prothrwo-Stith, D. (1996). Income distribution and mortality: Cross-sectional ecological study of the Robin Hood Index in the United States. *British Medical Journal, 312,* 1004–7.

43. Brown, L., Renner, M., & Flavin, C. (1997). *Vital signs.* New York: W. W. Norton.

44. Sapolsky, R. (1993); Sapolsky, R. (1994).

45. Sapolsky, R. (1994).

46. Marmot, M., & Theroll, T. (1988). Social class and cardiovascular disease: The contribution of work. *International Journal of Health Services, 18,* 659–74; Marmot, M. (1986). Social inequalities in mortality: The social environment. In R. Wilkinson (Ed.), *Class and health: Research and longitudinal data* (pp. 21–33). London: Tavistock; Marmot, M., Rose, G., Shipley, M., & Hamilton, P. (1978). Employment grade and coronary heart disease in British civil servants. *Journal of Epidemiology and Community Health, 32,* 244–49. For a more general discussion of psychosocial factors, see Evans, R., Barer, M., & Marmot, T. (Eds.). (1994).

47. Catalano, R., & Hartig, T. (2001). Communal bereavement and the incidence of very low birth weight in Sweden. *Journal of Health and Social Behavior, 42,* 333–41; Hedegaard, M., Henriksen, T., Secher, N., Hack, M., & Sabroe, S. (1996). Do stressful life events affect duration of gestation and risk of preterm delivery? *Epidemiology, 7,* 339–45; Hobel, C., Dunkel-Schetter, C., Roesch, S., Castro, L., & Arora, C. (1999). Maternal plasma corticotropin-releasing hormone associated with stress at 20 weeks' gestation in pregnancies ending in preterm delivery. *American Journal of Obstetrics and Gynecology, 180,* 257–64.; Lockwood, C. (1999). Stress-associated preterm delivery: The role of corticotropin-releasing hormone. *American Journal of Obstetrics and Gynecology, 180,* 264–66; Norbeck, J., DeJoseph, J., & Smith, R. (1996). A randomized trial of an empirically-driven social support intervention to prevent low birth weight among African American women. *Social Science and Medicine, 43,* 947–54.

48. Cooper, R., Goldenberg, R., Das, A., Elder, N., Swain, M., Norman, G., et al. (1996). The preterm prediction study: Maternal stress is associated with spontaneous preterm birth at less than thirty-five weeks' gestation. *American Journal of Obstetrics and Gynecology, 175,* 1286–92.

49. Hedegaard, M., Henriksen, T., Secher, N., Hack, M., & Sabroe, S. (1996); Lockwood, C. (1999).

50. Hobel, C., Dunkel-Schetter, C., Roesch, S., Castro, L., & Arora, C. (1999).

51. Sherraden, M., & Rossand, B. (1996). Poverty, family support and well-being of infants: Mexican immigrant women and child bearing. *Journal of Sociology and Social Welfare, 23(2),* 27–54.

52. Link, B. (1995), p. 84.

53. Link, B. (1995), p. 86.

54. Ernster, V. (1988). Trends in smoking, cancer risk, and cigarette promotion. *Cancer, 62,* 1702–12; Norton, T., Kenneth, E., Juliette, K., & Remington,

P. (1988). Smoking by blacks and whites: Socioeconomic and demographic differences. *American Journal of Public Health, 78,* 1187–89.

55. Judge, K. (1995). Income distribution and life expectancy. *British Medical Journal, 311,* 1282–85; Saunder, P. (1996). *Poverty, income distribution and health: An Australian study* (SPRC Reports and Proceedings No. 128). Sydney: University of New South Wales, Social Policy Research Center.

56. Gravelle, H. (1998). How much of the relationship between population mortality and unequal distribution of income is a statistical artifact. *British Medical Journal, 316,* 382–85; Friscella, K., & Franks, P. (1997). Poverty or income inequality as a predictor of mortality: Longitudinal cohort study. *British Medical Journal, 314,* 1724–28.

57. Kennedy, B., Kwachi, I., Glass, I., & Prothrow-Stith, D. (1998). Income distribution, socioeconomic status, and self-rated health: A U.S. multi-level analysis. *British Medical Journal, 317,* 917–21; Soobader, M., & LeClere, F. (1999). Aggregation and the measurement of income inequality: Effects on morbidity. *Social Science and Medicine, 48,* 733–44; Lochner, K. (1999). State inequality and individual mortality risk: A prospective multi-level study. Unpublished doctoral dissertation, Harvard University, Cambridge, MA.

58. Schneck, M., Sideras, K., Fox, R., & Dupuis, L. (1990). Low-income pregnancy, adolescents, and their infants: Dietary findings and health outcomes. *Journal of the American Dietetic Association, 90(4),* 555–58; Binsacca, D., Ellis, J., Martin, D., & Petitti, D. (1987). Factors associated with low birth-weight in an inner-city population: The role of financial problems. *American Journal of Public Health, 77,* 505–6; Lieberman, E., Ryan, K., Monson, R., & Schoenbaum, S. (1987).

59. Ounsted, M., & Scott, A. (1982). Social class and birthwieght: A new look. *Human Development, 6,* 83–89. For a discussion of the effects of gynecologic age, see Strobino, D., Ensminger, M., Kim, Y., & Nanda, J. (1995). Mechanisms for maternal age differences in birth weight. *American Journal of Epidemiology, 142,* 504–14.

60. Naeye, R. (1981). Teenaged and pre-teenaged pregnancies: Consequences of the fetal-maternal competition for nutrients. *Pediatrics, 67,* 146–50.

61. Scholl, T., Hediger, M., & Vasilenko, P. (1989). Effects of early maturation of fetal growth. *Annual Human Biology, 16,* 335–45.

62. Strobino, D., Ensminger, M., Kim, Y., & Nanda, J. (1995); Geronimus, A., & Korenman, S. (1993). Maternal youth or family background? On the health disadvantage of infants with teenage mothers. *American Journal of Epidemiology, 137,* 213–25.

63. Geronimus, A., Bound, J., Waidmann, T., Hillereier, M., & Burns, P. (1996). Excess mortality among blacks and whites in the United States. *New England Journal of Medicine, 335,* 1552–58.

64. Murphy, S. (2000).

65. Geronimus, A. (1997). Teenage childbearing and personal responsibility: An alternative view. *Political Science Quarterly, 112,* 405–30.

66. Starfield, B., Shapiro, S., Weiss, J., Liang, K., Ra, K., Paige, D., et al. (1991).

67. In our first model, shown in Table 3.3 in appendix B, we see that birth weight, on the whole, is quite insensitive to variations in income. The fixed-effects model also seems to indicate that income bears no relation to birth weight.

68. Due to small sample size, we could not isolate the effect for only those children of low-birth-weight mothers.

69. Reed, D., & Stanley, F. (Eds.). (1977); Kramer, M., Platt, R., Yang, H., McNamara, H., & Usher, R. (1999); Kallan, J. (1993).

70. Illsley, R. (1955); Gortmaker, S. (1979); Duncan, G., & Laren, D. (1990, February 13).

71. Baird, P. (1994). The role of genes in population health. In R. Evans, M. Barer, & T. Marmot (Eds.), *Why are some people healthy and others not?* (p. 136). New York: Aldine De Gruyter.

CHAPTER 4

1. Bennett, F. (1997).
2. Blakemore, B. (2000, July 5). An ethical dilemma. Retrieved July 15, 2000, from http://www.abcnews.com. For a further discussion see: Gross, R., Spiker, D., & Haynes, C. (Eds.). (1997); Hack, M., Flannery, D., Schluchter, M., Cartar, L., Borawski, E., & Klein, N. (2002).
3. Blakemore, B. (2000, July 5).
4. Collins, M., Halsey, C., & Anderson, C. (1991). Emerging development sequelae in the 'normal' extremely low birth weight infant. *Pediatrics, 88,* 115–20; Hagberg, B., Hagberg, G., Olow, I., & Von Wendt, L. (1989). The changing panorama of cerebral palsy in Sweden: The birth year period 1979–1982. *Acta Pediatrica Scandinavia, 78,* 283–90; Leonard, C., Clyman, R., Piecuch, R., Piecuch, R., Juster, R., & Ballard, R. (1990). Effect of medical and social risk factors on outcome of prematurity and very low birth weight. *Journal of Pediatrics, 116,* 620–26.
5. For a review of this literature, see Bennett, F. (1997).
6. For a review of this literature, see Bennett, F. (1997).
7. Klebanov, P. (1994). Classroom behavior of very low birth weight elementary school children. *Pediatrics, 94,* 700–8; Hack, M., Flannery, D., Schluchter, M., Cartar, L., Borawski, E., & Klein, N. (2002); Byrd, R., & Weitzman, M. (1994). Predictors of early grade retention among children in the United States. *Pediatrics, 93,* 481–87.
8. Sorensen, H., Sabroe, S., Olsen, J., Rothman, K., Gillman, M., & Fischer, P. (1997).
9. Strauss, R. (2000). Adult functional outcome of those born small for gestational age: Twenty-six-year follow-up of the 1970 British birth cohort. *Journal of the American Medical Association, 283,* 625–31.
10. Hack, M., Flannery, D., Schluchter, M., Cartar, L., Borawski, E., & Klein, N. (2002).
11. Rich-Edwards, J. (1997). Birth weight and risk of cardiovascular disease in a cohort of women followed-up since 1976. *British Medical Journal, 35,* 396–400.

12. Cameron, S., & Heckman, J. (1993). The nonequivalence of high school equivalents. *Journal of Labor Economics, 11,* 1–47; Horn, L., & Carroll, C. (1996). *Nontraditional undergraduates: Trends in enrollment from 1986 to 1992 and persistence and attainment among 1989–90 beginning postsecondary students* (Statistical Analysis Report No. 97578). Washington, DC: National Center for Education Statistics.

13. Hack, M., Klein, N., & Flannery, D. (2002). Correspondence: Outcomes in young adulthood for very-low-birth-weight infants: The authors reply. *New England Journal of Medicine, 347,* 142.

14. Bennett, F. (1988). Neurodevelopmental outcomes in low birthweight infants: The role of developmental intervention. In R. Guthrie (Ed.), *Neonatal intensive care: Clinics in critical care medicine* (pp. 221–50). New York: Churchill Livingstone.

15. McCormick, M., Shapiro, S., & Starfield, B. (1980).

16. McCormick, M., Stemmler, M., Bernbaum, J., & Ferran, A. (1986).

17. Tekolste, K., & Bennett, F. (1987).

18. Tekolste, K., & Bennett, F. (1987).

19. Bennett, F. (1997).

20. For a review of this research, see Gross, R., Spiker, D., & Haynes, C. (Eds.). (1997).

21. Scott, D., & Spiker, D. (1989); Rose. S. (1983). Differential rates of visual informational processing in full-term and pre-term infants. *Child Development, 54,* 11989–98.

22. Ruff, H., McCarton, C., Kurtzber, D., & Vaughan, H. (1984). Preterm infants' manipulative exploration of objects. *Child Development, 55,* 116–73.

23. McDonal, M., Sigma, M., & Ungerer, J. (1989). Intelligence and behavioral problems in 5-year-olds in relation to representational abilities in the second year of life. *Journal of Developmental Behavioral Pediatrics, 10,* 86–91.

24. McBurney, A., & Eaves, L. (1986). Evolution of developmental and psychological test scores. In H. Dunn (Ed.), *Sequelae of low birthweight: The Vancouver Study* (pp. 54–67). Philadelphia: Lippincott.

25. Wiener, G., Rider, R., Oppel, W., & Harper, P. (1968). Correlates of low birthweight: Psychological status at eight to ten years of age. *Pediatric Residence, 2,* 110.

26. Friedman, S., Jacobs, B., & Weithmann, M. (1982).

27. Spiker, D., Ferguson, J., & Brooks-Gunn, J. (1993). Enhancing maternal interactive behavior and child social competence in low birth weight, preterm infants. *Child Development, 64,* 754–86.

28. Escalona, S. (1987). *Critical issues in the early development of premature infants.* New Haven, CT: Yale University Press.

29. For a discussion of this literature, see Aber, J., Bennett, N., Conley, D., & Li, J. (1997).

30. Montgomery, S., Bartley, M., Cook, D., & Wadsworth, M. (1996). Health and social precursors of unemployment in young men. *Journal of Epidemiology and Community Health, 50,* 415–22.

31. For a discussion of these associations, see Wilkinson, R. (1996). *Unhealthy societies: The afflictions of inequality* (pp. 197–207). New York: Rout-

ledge; Wilkinson, R. (Ed.). (1986). *Class and health: Research and longitudinal data*. London: Tavistock.

32. Behrman, J., & Rosenzweig, M. (2001).

33. Steckel, R. (1983). Height and per capita income. *Historical Methods*, 16, 1–7.

34. Haines, M., Craig, L., & Weiss, T. (2000). *Development, health, nutrition, and mortality: The case of the 'antebellum puzzle' in the United States* (Historical Paper 130). Cambridge, MA: National Bureau of Economic Research; Martorell, R., & Habichit, J. P. (1986). Growth in early childhood in developing countries. In F. Faulkner & J. M. Tanner (Eds.), *Human growth: A comprehensive treatise, vol. 3* (pp. 241–62). New York: Plenum Press.

35. Korenman, S., & Miller, J. (1997). Effects of long-term poverty on physical health of children in the National Longitudinal Study of Youth. In G. Duncan & J. Brooks-Gunn (Eds.), *Consequences of growing up poor* (pp. 70–99). New York: Russell Sage Foundation.

36. Nystrom-Peck, M., & Lundberg, O. (1995). Short stature as an effect of economic and social conditions in childhood. *Social Science and Medicine, 41*, 733–38.

37. Montgomery, S., Bartley, M., & Wilkinson, R. (1997). Family conflict and slow growth. *Archive of Diseases in Children, 77*, 326–30.

38. For a general summary, see Aber, J., Bennett, N., Conley, D., & Li, J. (1997); Duncan, G., & Brooks-Gunn, J. (Eds.). (1997).

39. Smith, J., Brooks-Gunn, J., & Klebanov, P. (1997). Consequences of living in poverty for young children's cognitive and verbal ability and early school achievement. In G. Duncan & J. Brooks-Gunn (Eds.), *Consequences of growing up poor* (pp. 132–89). New York: Russell Sage Foundation.

40. See, for a review, Aber, J., Bennett, N., Conley, D., & Li, J. (1997).

41. For a review of this literature, see Aber, J., Bennett, N., Conley, D., & Li, J. (1997); Brooks-Gunn, J., Duncan, G., & Maritato, N. (1997). Poor families, poor outcomes: The well-being of children. In G. Duncan & J. Brooks-Gunn. (Eds.), *Consequences of growing up poor* (pp. 1–17). New York: Russell Sage Foundation; Hanson, T., McLanahan, S., & Thomson, E. (1997). Economic resources, parent practices, and children's well-being. In G. Duncan & J. Brooks-Gunn (Eds.), *Consequences of growing up poor* (pp. 190–238). New York: Russell Sage Foundation.

42. Hanson, T., McLanahan, S., & Thomson, E. (1997); Zill, N., Moore, K., Smith, E., Stief, T., & Corio, M. (1991).*The life circumstances and development on children in welfare families: A profile based on national survey data*. Washington, DC: Child Trends; Aber, J., Bennett, N., Conley, D., & Li, J. (1997).

43. Howes, C., & Stewart, P. (1987). Child's play with adults, toys, and peers: An examination of family and child care influences. *Developmental Psychology, 23*, 423–30; Howes, C., & Olenick, M. (1986). Family and child influences on toddlers' compliance. *Child Development, 26*, 292–303; Phillips, D., McCartney, K., & Scarr, S. (1987). Child care quality and children's social development. *Developmental Psychology, 23*, 537–43.

44. Conger, R., Conger, K., Elder, G., Lorenz, F., Simons, R., & Whitbeck, L. (1992). A family process model of economic hardship and adjustment of early

adolescent boys. *Child Development, 63*, 526–41; Conger, R., Ge, X., Elder, G., Lorenz, F., & Simons, R. (1994). Economic stress, coercive family process and developmental problems of adolescence. *Child Development, 65*, 541–61; Elder, G., Van Nguyen, T., & Caspi, A. (1995). Linking family hardship to children's lives. *Child Development, 56*, 361–75.

45. Conger, R., Ge, X., Elder, G., Lorenz, F., & Simons, R. (1994).

46. Duncan, G., & Brooks-Gunn, J. (1997).

47. For a review of this literature, see Starfield, B. (1991). Childhood morbidity: Comparisons, clusters, and trends. *Pediatrics, 88*, 519–26; Aber, J., Bennett, N., Conley, D., & Li, J. (1997).

48. Centers for Disease Control, National Center for Environmental Health. (n.d.); Centers for Disease Control, National Center for Environmental Health. (2001, December 22). Blood lead levels in young children: United States and selected states, 1996–1999. *Morbidity and Mortality Weekly Report, 49(50)*, 1133–37. Retrieved January 12, 2002, from http://www.cdc.gov/mmwr /preview/mmwr/html/mm4950a3.htm; Centers for Disease Control, National Center for Environmental Health. (n.d.). Asthma control programs and activities related to children and adolescents: Reducing costs and improving quality of life. Retrieved January 12, 2002, from http://www.cdc.gov/nceh /airpollution/asthma/children.htm

49. St. Peter, R., Newacheck, P., & Halfon, N. (1992). Access to care for poor children: Separate and unequal? *Journal of the American Medical Association, 267*, 2760–64.

50. Mayer, S. (1997). *What money can't buy: Family income and children's life chances*. Cambridge, MA: Harvard University Press.

51. Bradley, R., Whiteside, L., Mundform, D., Casey, P., Kehleher, K., & Pope, S. (1994); Parker, S., Greer, S., & Zuckerman, B. (1988). Double jeopardy: The impact of poverty on early child development. *Pediatric Clinics of North America, 35(6)*, 1227–40.

52. For a general review of the literature, see Aber, J., Bennett, N., Conley, D., & Li, J. (1997).

53. McGauhery, P. (1991). Social environment and vulnerability of low birth weight children: A social-epidemiological perspective. *Pediatrics, 88*, 943–53.

54. For a review, see Gross, R., Spiker, D., & Haynes, C. (Eds.). (1997).

55. Ramey, C., Bryant, D., Wasik, B., Sparling, J., Fendt, K., & Ange, L. (1992). Infant Health and Development Program for low birth weight, premature infants: Program elements, family participation, and child intelligence. *Pediatrics, 89*, 454–65.

56. Ramey, C., Bryant, D., Wasik, B., Sparling, J., Fendt, K., & Ange, L. (1992); McCormick, M., Workman-Daniels, K., & Brooks-Gunn, J. (1996). The behavioral and emotional well-being of school-age children with different birth weights. *Pediatrics, 97*, 18–25.

57. Pope, S. Whiteside, L., Brooks-Gunn, J., Kelleher, K., Rickert, V., Bradley, R., & Casey, P. (1993). Low-birth-weight infants born to adolescent mothers: Effects of co-residency with grandmother on child development. *Journal of the American Medical Association, 269*, 1319–1400.

58. For a review of this literature, see Aber, J., Bennett, N., Conley, D., & Li, J. (1997).

59. Brooks-Gunn, J., Gross, R., Kraemer, H., Spiker, D., & Shapiro, S. (1992). Enhancing the cognitive outcomes of low birth weight, premature infants: For whom is intervention most effective? *Pediatrics, 89,* 1209–15.

60. Cameron, S., & Heckman, J. (1993); Horn, L., & Carroll, C. (1996).

61. Duncan, G., & Brooks-Gunn, J. (1997); Duncan, G., Brooks-Gunn, J., Yeung, J., & Smith, J. (1998).

62. See appendix A for a further discussion of these variables.

63. See Table 4.4 in appendix B for these results.

64. See Table 4.4 in appendix B.

65. See appendix A for a further discussion of this data set.

66. Significant differences in birth weight are relatively common amongst twins, though the size of this difference varies in frequency. For instance, one study found that most twin pairs (72 percent of the sample) had birth weights within 15 percent of each other. Here the larger twin's birth weight is the standard for this percentage (or the denominator in the equation), so the smaller twin is 15 percent (or less) smaller than the larger twin. Fourteen percent of this sample had birth weight discordances between 15 and 20 percent, 7 percent had differences between 21 and 25 percent, 4 percent had differences between 26 and 30 percent, 3 percent had 31 to 40 percent discordance, and finally, 1 percent of the sample had birth weight differences exceeding 40 percent (Hollier, L., McIntire, D., & Leveno, K. [1999]. Outcome of twin pregnancies according to interpair birth weight differences. *Obstetrics and Gynecology, 94(6),* 1006–10.) Existing evidence seems to suggest that discordance of 30 percent or higher marks a significant threshold in the threat on birth outcomes. This implies that once one twin is about a third smaller than the other, there is a marked increase in the risks faced by the twin pair as a whole (Yalcin, H., Zorlu, C., Lembet, A., Ozden, S., & Gokmen, O. [1998]. The significance of birth weight difference in discordant twins: A level to standardize? *Acta Obstetrica Gyneologica Scandinavia, 77,* 28–31; Cheung, V., Bocking, A., & Dasilva, O. [1995]. Preterm discordant twins: What birth weight is significant? *American Journal of Obstetric Gynecology, 172,* 955–59; Hollier, L., McIntire, D., & Leveno, K. [1999]).

Given that birth weight has an effect on each individual twin's infant health, we would expect to consistently find that the smaller twin in a pair is significantly worse off than his or her larger counterpart. But results around this question are not consistent. Some studies have found no difference by size in the risk of morbidity (i.e., respiratory distress, intensive care admissions, seizures, etc.) or of mortality (i.e., fetal death and neonatal death) faced by twins in a given pair (Hollier, L., McIntire, D., & Leveno, K. [1999]; Talbot, G., Goldstein, R., Nesbitt, T., Johnson, J., & Kay, H. [1997]. Is size discordancy an indication for delivery of preterm twins? *American Journal of Obstetric Gynecology, 177,* 1050–54). Another study, however, has found that the smaller infant in a twin pair faces significantly higher risk of infant death when discordancy reaches 30 percent or higher (Cheung, V., Bocking, A., & Dasilva, O. [1995]). Still, another study found that there was no difference in respiratory distress between smaller and larger twins in twin pairs until gestation reached 28 weeks or more, at which point the heavier twin was more likely to need a respirator at four hours of age (although these authors caution that size appears to be less of a risk factor for respiratory distress than birth order and sex) (Webb, R., & Shaw, N. [2001]. Respiratory distress in heavier versus lighter twins. *Journal of Perinatal Medicine, 29,* 60–63). All of these studies are based on selective samples, however, which leaves open questions of generalizability. Webb, R., & Shaw, N. (2001) use a retrospective study of twin pairs under 36 weeks' gestation admitted to a regional neonatal unit over a three-year period. Cheung et al. (1995) study 122 live-born twin sets delivered between 25 and 34 weeks' gestation. Hollier et al. (1999) study 1,370 consecutive women who delivered at Parkland Hospital in Texas between January 1, 1996, and December 31, 1996. Talbot et al. (1997) have a retrospective study of hospital records of twins delivered between January 1, 1988, and June 30, 1995.

There is some evidence to suggest that these ambiguities have to do with gestational age. Twins with sizable discordance in growth rates represent a subsample of very-high-risk pregnancies. This implies that in many cases growth rate discordance is associated with preterm delivery (both spontaneous and induced). According to one study, physicians will often induce preterm labor in highly discordant twin pairs in order to reduce the risk of fetal death of the smaller twin (which causes even further complications for the surviving twin), but this tendency leads to alternative complications for the twin pair resulting from prematurity (Hollier, L., McIntire, D., & Leveno, K. [1999]). In short, because twins who are highly discordant are more likely to be delivered preterm, they face an increased risk of complications resulting from prematurity, which may overwhelm and obscure distinctions based on size. It should also be noted, though, that these studies that come to mixed results with respect to outcome differences by size among twin pairs generally do not take zygosity into account.

67. There is one study that separates out the effect of weight on risk of death by zygosity (West, C., Adi, Y., & Pharoah, P. [1999]. Fetal and infant death in mono- and dizygotic twins in England and Wales, 1982–1991. *Archive of Diseases in Childhood Fetal and Neonatal Edition, 80,* F217–F220). While this study finds a significant negative association between birth weight and infant mortality for twins, it does not use fixed-effects models. This means that, while this study tells us that low birth weight is important to the risk for infant mortality for individual twins (net of zygosity), it does not tell us how differences in birth weight in twin pairs matter (net of zygosity). Because this study does not use twin pair comparisons as we do, it cannot control for several factors that vary across pregnancies—including the important factor discussed above of prematurity in discordant twin pairs.

68. Odds of having twins and higher. (n.d.). Retrieved April 16, 2002, from http://www.geocities.com/factsaboutmultiples/twinbasics2.html

69. National Organization of Mothers of Twins Clubs, Inc. (n.d.). Twinning facts. Retrieved April 20, 2002, from http://www.nomotc.org/twinning _facts.html

70. Odds of having twins and higher. (n.d.).

71. Odds of having twins and higher. (n.d.).

72. National Organization of Mothers of Twins Clubs, Inc. (n.d.).

73. Martin, J., & Park, M. (1999). Trends in twin and triplet births: 1980–97. *National Vital Statistics Report, 47.* Hyattsville, MA: National Center for Health Statistics.

74. Centers for Disease Control, National Center for Health Statistics. (1999, September 14). Multiple birth rate for older women is sky rocketing (news release). Retrieved May 5, 2002, from http://www.cdc.gov/nchs/releases /99facts/multiple.htm

75. Martin, J., & Park, M. (1999).

76. West, C., Adi, Y., & Pharoah, P. (1999).

77. Parents' Place. (n.d.). Twin biology: Chorionicity of the placenta. Retrieved May 5, 2002, from http://www.parentsplace.com/pregnancy/labor /articles/0,10335,166530_111532,00.html

78. See, for instance, West, C., Adi, Y., & Pharoah, P. (1999); Hollier, L., McIntire, D., & Leveno, K. (1999).

79. Parents' Place. (n.d.).

80. Power, W., & Kiely, J. (1994). The risks confronting twins: A national perspective. *American Journal of Obstetrics and Gynecology, 170,* 456–61.

81. Williams, M., & O'Brien, W. (1997). Twins, asymmetric growth restriction, and perinatal morbidity. *Journal of Perinatology, 17,* 468–72.

CHAPTER 5

1. Health Care Financing Administration. (2000). Medicaid eligibility. Retrieved August 15, 2001, from http://www.hcfa.gov/medicaid/medicaid.htm

2. Toner, R. (2002, February 1). Administration plans care of fetuses in a health plan. [Electronic version]. *New York Times.* Retrieved February 1, 2002, from http://www.nytimes.com

3. Toner, R. (2002, February 1).

4. National Governors' Association. (1995, September). State Medicaid coverage of pregnant women and children. *MCH Update.* Washington, DC: Author.

5. Health Care Financing Administration. (2000).

6. Health Care Financing Administration. (2002). Special Medicaid coverage for pregnant women. Retrieved March 11, 2002, from http://www.hcfa .gov/hiv/subpg4.htm

7. Health Care Financing Administration. (2000).

8. Specifically, Connecticut, Delaware, Florida, Hawaii, Iowa, Kentucky, Maine, Maryland, Massachusetts, Michigan, Mississippi, Missouri, New Hampshire, New Jersey, New York, North Carolina, Oklahoma, Pennsylvania, South Carolina, Tennessee, Washington, and Wisconsin have opted to use high cutoffs.

9. Health Care Financing Administration. (2002).

10. Still, these most recent Medicaid eligibility standards for pregnant women are something of an improvement over previous standards. Prior to the mid-1980s, pregnant women had to be living below the poverty line in order to be eligible for benefits—that is, the income cutoff was set at 100 percent of the

poverty line rather than the current 133 percent. In the latter half of the 1980s, however, concern over high infant mortality rates grew, and Medicaid eligibility standards were correspondingly expanded to include more pregnant women. In just six years, from 1984 to 1990, Congress amended Medicaid ten times, altering the program to offer further coverage to pregnant women and young children (Coughlin, T., Ku, L., & Holahan, J. [1994]. *Medicaid since the 1980s: Costs, coverage, and the shifting alliance between the federal government and the states* (pp. 47–61). Washington, DC: Urban Institute Press.). These recent revisions certainly helped reduce gaps in coverage for pregnant women that had previously resulted from low income eligibility levels. Prior to the mid-1980s, members of the near-poor and working poor generally did not qualify for Medicaid, which meant they were chronically uninsured, since employer-sponsored insurance is also generally lacking in this group.

These changes in eligibility standards can be fit within a larger historical problem of periodic cuts in Medicaid spending. Medicaid is a federal matching grants program, meaning that the federal government reimburses states for portions of the Medicaid costs that they have incurred over the past fiscal period. This "after-the-fact" payment implies that the only way for Congress to control the costs of the program is to cut back the program itself. (For a discussion of this dilemma, see Stevens, R., & Stevens, R. [1974].) If Congress were to set the Medicaid budget before the fiscal period, states would be forced to work within particular financial confines. As the program currently stands, however, the federal government is given almost no influence or leverage before costs are incurred and, thus, can only limit states' spending by amending the program's eligibility standards. Rather unsurprisingly, this structure has meant that Medicaid is very vulnerable to cuts and reductions in eligibility standards. The historical pattern of Medicaid spending is generally such that, when the economy is relatively strong and state and federal governments have balanced budgets, Medicaid seems to thrive. However, when the economy turns and budgets can no longer be so easily reconciled, Medicaid is frequently one of the first social programs to be cut. This tendency often places the poor in double jeopardy—under slow economic conditions, when the poor are particularly in need of public assistance because the private sphere is usually suffering, public assistance is highly likely to be cut. Indeed, prior to the expansion of eligibility criteria in the late 1980s, Medicaid had been severely slashed, leaving many of the poor without health insurance.

11. Health Care Financing Administration. (2000).

12. U.S. Department of Agriculture. (n.d.). WIC income eligibility criteria, 2001–2002. Retrieved September 20, 2001, from http://www.fns.usda.gov/wic/incomeeligguidelines02-03.htm

13. Persons participating in Temporary Assistance for Needy Families (TANF) and the Food Stamps program are also automatically eligible for WIC.

14. U.S. Department of Agriculture. (n.d.).

15. U.S. Department of Agriculture. (2000). *WIC participant and program characteristics, 1998* (Nutrition Assistance Program Report Series, Special Nutrition Programs, Report No. WIC-00-PC: 67–72). [Electronic Version]. Washington. DC: Author. Retrieved September 23, 2001, from http://www.fns.usda.gov/oane/MENU/Published/WIC/WIC.htm

16. For a review of this literature, see Moss, N., & Carver, K. (1998); Avruch, S., & Cackley, A. (1995); Widga, A., & Lewis, N. (1999); Buescher, P., Larson, L., & Lenihan, A. (1993). Prenatal WIC participation can reduce low birth weight and newborn medical costs: A cost benefit analysis of WIC participation in North Carolina. *Journal of the American Dietetic Association, 93,* 163–66.

17. Avruch, S., & Cackley, A. (1995).

18. U.S. Department of Agriculture. (2000). *WIC participant and program characteristics, 1998,* pp. 149–53.

19. These data are available only for 1998 because it was in this year that the federal government sponsored a study of the costs associated with Medicaid prenatal care. See U.S. General Accounting Office. (1998, May). *Medicaid prenatal care: States improve access and enhance services but face new challenges.* Washington, DC: U.S. Government Printing Office.

20. U.S. General Accounting Office (1994, May).

21. U.S. General Accounting Office (1994, May); U.S. Department of Agriculture. (1990, October). *The savings in Medicaid costs for newborns and their mothers from prenatal participation in the WIC program, Volume 1.* [Electronic Version]. Washington, DC: U.S. Government Printing Office. Retrieved October 2, 2001, from http://www.fns.usda.gov/oane/MENU/Published/WIC /WIC.htm.; U.S. Department of Agriculture. (1991, October). *The savings in Medicaid costs for newborns and their mothers from prenatal participation in the WIC program, Addendum.* [Electronic Version]. Washington, DC: U.S. Government Printing Office. Retrieved October 2, 2001, from http://www.fns .usda.gov/oane/MENU/Published/WIC/WIC.htm; U.S. Department of Agriculture. (1992, April). *The savings in Medicaid costs for newborns and their mothers from prenatal participation in the WIC program, Volume 2* [Electronic Version]. Washington, DC: U.S. Government Printing Office. Retrieved October 2, 2001, from http://www.fns.usda.gov/oane/MENU/Published/WIC/WIC .htm

22. Kallan, J. (1993).

23. State Policy Documentation Project. (1999). Categorical eligibility: Pregnant women. Retrieved March 20, 2002, from http://www.spdp.prg/tanf /categorical/pregwom.pdf

24. State Policy Documentation Project. (1999). Financial eligibility for TANF cash assistance. Retrieved March 20, 2002, from http://www.spdp .org/tanf/financial/finansumm.htm

25. State Policy Documentation Project. (1999). Financial eligibility for TANF cash assistance; Coven, M. (2002, February 14). *An introduction to TANF* (Center on Budget and Policy Priorities Policy Report). [Electronic Version]. Washington, DC: Center on Budget and Policy Priorities. Retrieved March 20, 2002, from http://www.cbpp.org/1-22-02tanf2.pdf

26. State Policy Documentation Project. (1999). Financial eligibility for TANF cash assistance.

27. For a discussion of family cap policies, see Weaver, R. (2000). *Ending welfare as we know it.* Washington, DC: Brookings Institution Press, chapter 13.

28. For a review of this research, see Weaver, R. (2000), chapter 6.

29. There are some further issues surrounding TANF that warrant mention. The young TANF program, established with the 1996 Personal Responsibility and Work Opportunity Reconciliation Act (PRWORA), has imposed further, unprecedented and controversial restrictions on eligibility. For instance, under TANF the federal government can impose time limits on assistance. Since 1996 states have been unable to use federal TANF block grant funds to provide more than a cumulative lifetime total of 60 months of cash assistance to any welfare recipient. Women simply become ineligible for assistance once this 60-month period is reached (Administration for Children and Families. [2002]. Fact sheets: Welfare: Temporary Assistance for Needy Families. Retrieved August 15, 2001, from http://www.acf.dhhs.gov/news/facts/tanf.html).

Work requirements are another controversial part of the 1996 TANF legislation. Since 1996, single parents with no child under a given age (which varies by state) have been required to work or participate in work-related activities (such as vocational training) at least 30 hours per week in order to maintain eligibility for cash assistance (State Policy Documentation Project. [2000]. State policies regarding TANF work activities and requirements. Retrieved March 20, 2002, from http://www.spdp.org/tanf/sanctions/sanctions_findings.htm). In cases of disability or other exceptional circumstances, states can grant exceptions to the lifetime limit and work requirements and continue to use federal funds for up to 20 percent of their caseload. There is evidence to suggest, however, that this 20 percent limit significantly underestimates the number of women who cannot work because of their own or their child's disabilities (Polit, D., London, A., & Martinez, J. [2001, May]. *The health of poor urban women: Findings from the Project on Devolution and Urban Change* (Manpower Demonstration Research Corporation Report). [Electronic Version]. New York: Manpower Demonstration Research Corporation. Retrieved October 10, 2001, from http://www.mdrc.org/Publications.htm). The legislation surrounding this 20 percent exception further does not take into account the possibility of economic slowdowns and decreased demand for less skilled workers. Thus, at times when the economy is weak and there is a reduced demand for unskilled labor, unemployed women who have reached time limits and are unable to find work because of a bad market may be left entirely without assistance.

This TANF program truly represents a sweeping change from prior cash assistance policy. In signing PRWORA into law in 1996, President Clinton vowed to "do away with welfare as we know it," and for all intents and purposes, he did. Before the 1996 reforms, cash assistance, know as Aid to Families with Dependent Children (AFDC), was a federal matching grants program that reimbursed states for cash assistance spending after the fiscal year had ended. Nor did earlier welfare policy contain provisions about time limits or work requirements, so eligibility standards were generally less stringent. AFDC's less stringent matching grants structure meant that enrollment levels and costs frequently rose and fell with the economic tides. But it also meant that, when the economy changed and unemployment rates rose, states could expand their cash assistance programs accordingly, avoiding large increases in poverty rates. Under TANF, with federal grants now set before the fiscal period begins, such options for expansion are essentially eliminated. Because spending is set at the 1994 level, increased welfare costs resulting from economic downturns or changes in the population will have to be carried by the states or, in states that do not have funds or inclinations to extend benefits, by the poor themselves (Coven. M. [2002, February 14]; Weaver, R. [2000]).

In many respects the late 1990s offered the young TANF program the ideal circumstances in which to prove itself. Since during this time, the economy was strong and unemployment low, it was easier than it had been in decades for welfare recipients to find jobs and conform to work requirements and time limits. Yet data available five years after reform, in 2001, suggest that results have been mixed despite a prosperous economy. At a superficial level it appears that reform attained it goals—the old welfare system was done away with in the sense that the rolls shrank and more recipients were working. However, when examining the situation more deeply, the story becomes less optimistic and significantly more mixed. On one hand, it appears that women who left welfare and were working are better off than their counterparts who remained on welfare. According to estimates by Sheldon Danziger, the average monthly income in 1998 for women who had left welfare and were working was $1,405, while those who were combining welfare and work were earning $1,277 and those who were wholly reliant on welfare were bringing in only $892. However, as Danziger also points out, there is a flip side of this story. Those who found work and were in the comparatively best situation still faced a 47.4 percent chance of living below the poverty line (Danziger, S. [2000]. *Approaching the limit: Early national lessons from welfare reform* (working paper). Ann Arbor, MI: University of Michigan, Poverty Research and Training Center). That is, even women who were employed in 1998, conforming to the goals of TANF, were encountering significant financial risk.

The story behind TANF's semisuccess becomes increasingly troubling when we consider in greater detail the shrinking of welfare rolls that supposedly marked the end of welfare as we knew it. Indeed, the diversity of those who left the welfare rolls has indicated to many analysts that not all those who exited welfare improved their situations. Some women who left the rolls had reasonable human capital, found jobs, and were supporting themselves in 1998. However, many of the women who left the rolls were among the rolls' most disadvantaged recipients and had not found employment by 1998 (National Center for Children in Poverty, Research Forum on Children, Families, and the New Federalism. [2001]. *Three-city findings reveal unexpected diversity among welfare leavers and stayers* [Research Report]. New York: Author; Danziger, S. [2000].). Evidence suggests that this minor exodus of disadvantaged recipients is likely the result of an increase use of sanctions against those who were the most disadvantaged. The 1996 welfare reform law allowed states to impose "full-family sanctions," which stop benefits completely if families are not following program rules. Researchers have suggested that three times as many families left welfare by 1998 because of such sanctions as left because they reached a time limit, and the most common reasons for being penalized were administrative—usually missing a meeting with a caseworker or failing to file paperwork. Further, researchers have found that those who were sanctioned in such a way generally had less education, were in poorer health, lived in poor quality housing, and had lower monthly incomes than those who had not been sanctioned (National Center for Children in Poverty, Research Forum on Children, Families, and the New Federalism. [2001]). Such individuals are, unsurprisingly, relatively unlikely to find good employment once off welfare, so sanctioned individuals were bringing in an average monthly income of only $798 in 1998 and were facing a 78.6 percent chance of living below the poverty line (Danziger, S. [2000].).

The 1996 welfare reform law has raised several complicated issues. Even today, in 2002, it remains quite unclear what the reform's ultimate effect will be. Data are still coming in, and it remains to be seen what will happen as more recipients begin to reach time limits. Changes in general economic conditions may also have severe effects on the welfare population, given work requirements, and it remains unclear what will happen during economic lags.

30. Internal Revenue Service. (2002). EITC overview. Retrieved October 5, 2002, from www.irs.gov/ind_info/eitc-ovrvw.html

31. Internal Revenue Service. (2002). EITC overview.

32. Internal Revenue Service. (2002). Child Tax Credit: Topic 606. Retrieved October 5, 2002, from www.irs.gov/tax_edu/teletax/tc606.html

33. Internal Revenue Service. (2002). Child Tax Credit: Topic 606.

34. Internal Revenue Service. (2002). Child Tax Credit: Topic 606.

35. Miscarriages may not actually be a very large practical concern here, since they tend to happen very early within a pregnancy. It would seem that, by the time a woman knows she is pregnant and files for reduced withholdings, she would most likely be past the stages during which the majority of miscarriages take place.

36. See, for instance, two classical works: Hunt, J. (1961). *Intelligence and experience.* New York: Ronald Press; Bloom, B. (1964). *Stability and change in human characteristics.* New York: John Wiley & Sons.

37. See, for example, Bennett, F. (1997); Collins, M., Halsey, C., & Anderson, C. (1991); Klebanov, P. (1994); Byrd, R., & Weitzman, M. (1994).

38. It should be noted that some authors do not attribute such an important role to income and consider parental characteristics (such as education, personality, or motivation) to be of greater influence on children's outcomes. For an example of this approach, see Mayer, S. (1997).

39. Administration for Children and Families. (2002); State Policy Documentation Project. (2000). State policies regarding TANF work activities and requirements.

40. State Policy Documentation Project. (2000). State policies regarding TANF work activities and requirements. Note that many states also have policies in which families with "good cause" for noncompliance with work requirements may avoid having a sanction imposed on the family. As of 2000, 37 out of 50 states include caring for a disabled family member to be a good-cause reason for noncompliance. Because these good-cause provisions, however, allow only temporary avoidance of sanctions, they may not be of much help when dealing with disabilities that are generally long term. For a further discussion of

states' good-cause provisions, see State Policy Documentation Project. (2000). Sanctions for non-compliance with work activities. Retrieved March 20, 2002, from http://www.spdp.org/tanf/sanctions.htm

41. U.S. Department of Agriculture. (2000). WIC general analysis project: Profile of WIC children. Retrieved September 23, 2001, from http://www.fns .usda.gov/oane/MENU/published/WIC/FILES/profile.pdf

42. Long, S., Kurka, R., Waters, S., & Kirby, G. (1998). *Child care assistance under welfare reform: Early responses by the states* (Assessing the New Federalism Series, Paper No. 15). [Electronic Version]. Washington, DC: Urban Institute Press. Retrieved September 27, 2002, from http://www.urban.org /Template.cfm?NavMenuID=24.

43. Long, S., Kurka, R., Waters, S., & Kirby, G. (1998).

44. For a brief discussion of this problem, see Long, S., Kurka, R., Waters, S., & Kirby, G. (1998).

45. Social Security Administration. (2002). SSI payment amounts, 1975–2002. Retrieved March 15, 2002, from http://www.ssa.gov/OACT/COLA /SSIamts.html

46. Social Security Administration. (2000). *Benefits for children with disabilities* (SSA publication No. 05-10026). [Electronic version]. Washington, DC: Author. Retrieved March 15, 2002, from www.ssa.gov/pubs/10026.html.

47. Loprest, P. (1997). *Supplemental security income for children with disabilities* (Issues and Options for States Series, Paper No. A-10). [Electronic version]. Washington, DC: Urban Institute Press. Retrieved March 15, 2002, http://www.urban.org/Template.cfm?NavMenuID=24

48. Loprest, P. (1997).

49. Loprest, P. (1997).

50. While cash assistance is obviously helpful when trying to increase the resources available to low-birth-weight children, it alone cannot provide access to basic necessities. In-kind benefits may be very important in supplementing these cash assistance programs.

Medicaid is a crucial program in this discussion as it provides health insurance to the vast majority of low-income children. In 1994–1995, for instance, 48.5 percent of children living below 200 percent of the poverty line were covered by Medicaid (Liska, D., Brennan, N., & Bruen, B. [2001]. *State level databook on health care access and financing.* 3rd ed. Washington, DC: Urban Institute Press). This relatively high rate does not mean, however, that health insurance is available to all low-income children who might need it. Gaps remain in health insurance coverage for children. In particular, as children get older and as incomes approach the category of near-poor, we begin to see children who lack employer-based insurance falling through cracks in Medicaid eligibility.

Federal legislation greatly emphasizes providing health care to young children, and accordingly, we find that only low percentages—in 1995 only 6.1 percent—of poor children between the ages of one and five lack insurance. As income begins to increase, however, this rate also increases. The percentage of children ages one to five who are uninsured more than doubles—to over 15 percent—for those living in families with incomes between 135 and 185 percent of the poverty line. States are required to provide Medicaid to children between ages six and twelve, yet we still see the rate of uninsured for poor children rising to 9.9 percent as we reach this age group. The reasons for this increase are somewhat unclear perhaps because there is less of a legislative emphasis placed on this older group and because the program is not publicized as well for this population and therefore enrollment rates are lower. For the near-poor children (between 100 and 185 percent of the poverty line) in this age group, rates of uninsured are even higher, reaching 19 percent. As poor children approach ages 13 to 18, Medicaid coverage becomes optional at the federal level and therefore varies significantly by state. As a result, we find quite high rates—about one-fifth—of poor children between 13 and 18 are uninsured. Income plays a slightly smaller role for this group, since Medicaid is a less crucial insurance provider for this group. Indeed, near-poor teenagers between the ages of 13 and 18 face uninsured rates that are rather similar to those of poor teenagers— approximately 23 percent (Holahan, J. [1997]. *Expanding insurance coverage for children* (Policy Report). [Electronic version]. Washington, DC: Urban Institute Press. Retrieved March 20, 2002, from http://www.urban.org).

This general drop-off in insurance rates by age and income may be partially addressed by federal legislation implementing the State Child Health Insurance Program (SCHIP). The SCHIP legislation, passed in 1997, gave states the option of using Medicaid, a separate state program, or some combination of the two to expand coverage to low-income children. Under this legislation, almost all states have increased eligibility thresholds for children of all ages to at least 200 percent of the poverty line (Dubay, L. [2002]. *Children's eligibility for Medicaid and SCHIP: A view from 2002* [New Federalism: National Survey of America's Families Series, Policy Review Paper No. B-41]. [Electronic version]. Washington, DC: Urban Institute Press. Retrieved March 20, 2002, from http://www.urban.org). Despite this expansion, though, a recent study found that 22 percent of low-income children (those with family incomes below 200 percent of the poverty line) were still falling through the cracks and remained uninsured in 1999 (Liska, D., Brennan, N., & Bruen, B. (2001). This finding could have to do with disregards under SCHIP. Since most states' SCHIP programs allow less of a family's income to be disregarded in eligibility calculation than states' Medicaid programs allow, differences between Medicaid and SCHIP income standards are often less than they appear. Thus, near-poor children may fall through cracks in SCHIP just as they fall though cracks in Medicaid. While older children who are not covered under Medicaid may be more likely to be covered under SCHIP, children living close to, but not actually below, the poverty line may still be quite vulnerable. Low-birth-weight children, particularly those living in low-income households, suffer from poorer health *at all ages* as compared to normal-birth-weight children (Dubay, L. [2002]). These gaps in coverage that disproportionately affect the near-poor and older children are thus particularly troubling.

Another area in which direct assistance is an important supplement to cash assistance is diet. As discussed before, WIC provides supplementary food, nutrition education, and health care referrals to nutritionally at-risk pregnant women, infants, and children with low incomes. Most evidence suggests that

WIC does a good job at this and generally improves the nutritional status and health of child participants. However, WIC covers children only through age five and, once WIC's preset budget limits have been reached, children generally have lower priority status than pregnant women and infants. Since nutrition clearly matters to health and development beyond the WIC age-five cutoff, many families turn to Food Stamps for additional nutritional assistance. Food Stamps are a federal program that provides vouchers to help low-income families and individuals purchase nutritious low-cost meals. To participate in Food Stamps, householders must have a monthly income below 130 percent of the federal poverty line and no more than $2,000 in assets (as of 2001) (Social Security Administration. [1998]. *Food stamps and other nutritional programs.* [Publication No. 05-10100]. [Electronic version]. Washington, DC: Author. Retrieved September 25, 2001, from http://www.ssa.gov). Food stamps are often a crucial component of a poor family's income, and federal spending on Food Stamps has traditionally exceeded spending on other large programs, such as Medicaid and cash assistance (Gundersen, C., LeBlanc, M., & Kuhn, B. [1999]. *The changing food assistance landscape: The Food Stamp program in a post-welfare reform environment* [Agricultural Economics Report No. 773]. Washington, DC: U.S. Department of Agriculture, Economics Research Service). However, as has been the case with most of the programs we have discussed so far, the 1996 Welfare Reform Act significantly altered the legislation supporting this program. The 1996 reform bill cut more funds, through reductions in eligibility and benefits, from the Food Stamps program than from any other program. With the reform act, most legal immigrants became ineligible, leading to approximately a 7 percent drop in Food Stamps participation. Benefit levels for all participants also fell from an average of 80 cents per person per meal to 75 cents (Gundersen, C., LeBlanc, M., & Kuhn, B. [1999]).

Given the importance of nutrition to child development, such reductions can have an obvious impact on low-birth-weight children (and children more generally) by determining the quantity and quality of food families can buy. Beyond these direct effects, however, decreases in food stamp can also lead to lower expenditures for rent, clothing, and medical care as scarce resources are reallocated in the household (Gundersen, C., LeBlanc, M., & Kuhn, B. [1999]). So even reductions that are specifically limited to food stamps can have far-reaching implications, leading to higher levels of overall depravation.

51. For a review of these two programs, see Ramey, C., & Ramey, S. (1994). Which children benefit the most from early intervention? *Pediatrics, 94,* 1064–66.

52. Gross, R., Spiker, D., & Haynes, C. (Eds.). (1997). These low-birth-weight-specific intervention programs have generally taken a broad approach to the problem of education, paying particular attention to biosocial interactions and drawing on such frameworks as biosocial systems theory. In such broad approaches to early development, multiple influences are assumed to interact over time. Specifically, in the biosocial systems approach, it is hypothesized that the developmental progress of the child and the caregiver is the result of the biological and social historical contexts of the two, the influence of these factors on their current status, as well as potential future transactions among

the child, caregiver, and their environments. In an approach such as this, ample space is carved out for the complexities of human development.

For a discussion of biosocial systems theory, see Ramey, C., Sparling, J., Bryant, D., & Wasik, B. (1997). The intervention model. In R. Gross, D. Spiker, & C. Haynes (Eds.), *Helping low birth weight, premature babies: The Infant Health and Development Program* (pp. 17–26). Stanford, CA: Stanford University Press.

53. Gross, R. (1997). The primary child outcomes. In R. Gross, D. Spiker, & C. Haynes (Eds.), *Helping low birth weight, premature babies: The Infant Health and Development Program* (pp. 139–54). Stanford, CA: Stanford University Press.

54. Gross, R. (1997).

55. Brooks-Gunn, J., Gross, R., Kraemer, H., Spiker, D., & Shapiro, S. (1992).

56. Brooks-Gunn, J., Gross, R., Kraemer, H., Spiker, D., & Shapiro, S. (1992); Gross, R. (1997).

57. Brooks-Gunn, J., Gross, R., Kraemer, H., Spiker, D., & Shapiro, S. (1992).

58. U.S. Department of Education, Office of Special Education Programs. (2002). Individuals With Disabilities Education Act: Program-funded activities fiscal year 2001. Retrieved September 25, 2001, from http://www.ed.gov/offices/OSERS/OSEP/Programs/PFA2001/

59. U.S. Department of Education, Early Childhood Technical Assistance Center. (2002). Overview to the Part C Program under IDEA. Retrieved October 1, 2001, from http://www.ectac.org

60. SRI International. (1999). *National Early Intervention Longitudinal Study (NEILS): State-to-state variations in early intervention Systems* (Report prepared for the Office of Special Education Programs, U.S. Department of Education). Retrieved October 1, 2001, from http://www.sri.com/neils/reports.html

61. According to SRI International's report (1999), federal examples of conditions that are assumed to result in developmental delays include chromosomal abnormalities, genetic or congenital disorders, severe sensory impairments, inborn errors of metabolism, disorders reflecting disturbance of the nervous system's development, and disorders secondary to toxic exposure (including fetal alcohol syndrome).

62. It should be noted that a state's not including at-risk children in this program does not necessarily imply that the state provides no services for at-risk young children. States may provide these services through alternative local programs.

63. SRI International. (1999).

64. U.S. Department of Education. (1996). To assure the free appropriate public education of all children with disabilities: 18th annual report to Congress on the implementation of the Individuals with Disabilities Education Act. Retrieved October 1, 2001, from www.ed.gov/pubs/OSEP96AnlRpt/chap3.html

65. U.S. Department of Education. (1996).

66. U.S. Department of Education. (1996). Note that the remaining portion of children participating in this program is served in resource rooms, separate schools, residential facilities, or homes/hospitals.

67. U.S. Department of Education, Office of Special Education Programs. (2000). To assure the free appropriate public education of all children with disabilities: 22nd annual report to Congress on the implementation of the Individuals with Disabilities Education Act. Retrieved October 1, 2001, from http://www.ed.gov/offices/OSERS/OSEP/products/OSEP2000AnlRpt/index.hml

68. U.S. Department of Education, Office of Special Education Programs. (2000).

69. U.S. Department of Education, Office of Special Education Programs. (2000).

70. Washington, V., & Bailey, U. (1995). *Project Head Start: Models and strategies for the twenty-first century*. New York: Garland.

71. For a discussion of Head Start's structure, see Washington, V., & Bailey, U. (1995); Zigler, E., & Styfco, S. (1993). *Head Start and beyond: A national plan for extended childhood intervention*. New Haven, CT: Yale University Press.

72. Ramey, C., & Ramey, S. (1994).

73. U.S. Department of Education, Office of Special Education Programs. (2000).

74. Cicirelli, V. (1969). *The impact of Head Start: An evaluation of the effects of Head Start on children's cognitive and affective development* (Report No. PB 184 328, presented to the Office of Economic Opportunity). Washington, DC: Westinghouse Learning Corporation; Currie, J., & Thomas, D. (1995). Does Head Start make a difference? *American Economic Review, 85,* 341–64.

75. For a discussion of these issues, see Zigler, E., & Styfco, S. (1993).

76. Holden, C. (1990). Head Start enters adulthood. *Science, 247,* 1400.

77. There are five fundamental provision of special education outlined in the Individuals with Disabilities Education Act (IDEA). According to the first of these provisions, all students with special needs are guaranteed an Individualized Education Program (IEP) developed under the guidance of a team of parents and professionals. This IEP is expected to address such questions as long- and short-term goals, methods of assessment, and degree of participation in general education. Since there is much diversity in the types and severity of children's impairments, this guarantee of individualized services can be quite important. The second measure outlined in the act builds upon guarantees of individualized attention and requires that services be provided in the least restrictive environment. That is, students with special needs must be offered a wide variety of services, ranging from placement in the general education classroom to homebound instruction. This "cascade of services" guarantees that disabled students will be integrated, to the greatest degree possible and appropriate, into mainstream education. The third provision calls for nondiscriminatory testing and mandates that all contact with the learner, including evaluation, be conducted in the learner's native language. Early and correct diagnosis of a disability can be crucial to a child's success, but overzealousness can lead to

incorrect diagnoses, which can be quite harmful to children. This provision begins to address this problem, guaranteeing that children are tested in an appropriate manner so as to reduce the possibility of an inappropriate diagnosis. The fourth provision in IDEA provides for confidentiality of information and record keeping. And the act's fifth provision guarantees that the learner will not be evaluated or the education program altered until parental permission has been granted (Schloss, P., Smith, M., & Schloss, C. [2001]. *Instructional methods for secondary students with learning and behavioral problems* [3rd ed]. Boston: Allyn & Bacon).

78. Smith, D. (1998) *Introduction to special education: Teaching in an age of challenge* (3rd ed). Boston: Allyn & Bacon.

79. Smith, D. (1998), p. 51.

80. Smith, D. (1998), pp. 54–56.

81. Smith, D. (1998), p. 57.

82. Smith, D. (1998), pp. 59–61.

83. Smith, D. (1998), pp. 61–63.

84. There is not a great deal to say specifically about secondary special education, primarily because it is a poorly defined and often unattended-to area within special education. In line with the general emphasis placed on early ages in children's services, special education for older children is generally less comprehensive and appropriate than comparable services for younger children. Patrick Schloss and his colleagues, in reviewing the quality of special education for secondary students, write that "services available to secondary students may be little more than a repetition or a continuation of elementary-level programs. Special education teachers who are not specifically trained for work at this level may use instructional strategies that have not been validated for secondary learners. In addition, the instructional materials frequently used at this level may have been intended either for elementary students with disabilities or for secondary students who are not disabled" (Schloss, P., Smith, M., & Schloss, C. [2001], p. 3).

This poor quality of secondary special education can be linked to a general lack of recognition of the need for secondary special education in recent policy. For instance, the School-to-Work Opportunity Act, signed into law in 1994, was intended to reform secondary education in order to better prepare children for the labor market, yet it makes no mention of secondary students with special needs. Additional legislation around this time, such as the Goals 2000: Educate America Act, similarly addresses a broad collection of issues, ranging from parental participation to school safety, while making no mention of secondary special education (for a discussion of this legislation, see Schloss, P., Smith, M., & Schloss, C. [2001]). In other words, the importance of secondary special education has not been adequately realized in Washington, and therefore the funds, training, and research that would support this service are simply not available.

All the same, there are several reasons that high school students with impairments are in great need of services. Succeeding in high school may be particularly difficult for students with disabilities because the structure and curriculum in secondary education are generally more rigid, making fewer allowances for particular needs than those found in primary education. Unlike the elementary education in which students begin, the high school education system requires that students deal with several teachers over the course of a day, with a curriculum set around common standards and with a lecture format that may be less than ideal for many impaired students. Schloss and his colleagues, outline several reasons why impaired students may not bring to this learning situation all of the skills necessary for success. Among these reasons, they note that impaired students are less likely to acquire information and skills through experiences incidental to the learning task and are less able to generalize information and skills from one setting or condition to another (Schloss, P., Smith, M., & Schloss, C. [2001], p. 79.).

In addition to these specific learning issues, adolescence can also be a very troubling and turbulent time in the more general process of human development. During adolescence there are many critical decisions to be made and teenagers with impairments may have a great deal of trouble making rational choices about their future career prospects and life goals. Thus, in serving secondary students with disabilities, particular attention might also need to be paid to nonacademic issues such as juvenile delinquency, drug use, and sexually transmitted diseases (for a further discussion of these issues, see Schloss, P., Smith, M., & Schloss, C. [2001]).

Clearly the general state of secondary special education is a problem. For low-birth-weight children, who have a disproportionate need for special services in secondary education, this state is even more troubling. However, while recent policy has not adequately addressed the issue, there is some hope for the future. Recently, educational reform efforts have paid increased attention to the needs of secondary students with impairments through the provision of transition services. The Office of Special Education and Rehabilitation Services (OSERS) has developed a three-part definition of the transition period. According to this definition, transition is (i) a period that includes high school, the point of graduation, additional post-secondary education or adult services, and the initial years of employment; (ii) a process that requires sound preparation in the secondary school and adequate support at the point of school leaving; and (iii) an effort that emphasizes the shared responsibility of all involved parties for success (Will, M. [1984]. *Bridges from school to working life: OSERS programming for the transition of youth with disabilities* [policy report]. Washington DC: U.S. Department of Education, Office of Special Education and Rehabilitation Services, p. 2). Legislation since the early 1990s has begun to recognize this important period in young adults' lives. For instance, in 1990 an amendment to the Individuals with Disabilities Education Act mandated transition services for student's with disabilities, including career planning, postsecondary training, financial assistance, medical support, and insurance (for a discussion of this legislation, see Schloss, P., Smith, M., & Schloss, C. [2001], pp. 1–20.).

APPENDIX A

1. Hill, M. (1992). *The panel study of income dynamics: A user's guide.* Newbury Park, CA: Sage; Institute for Social Research, University of Michigan.

(2000, August). *An overview of the Panel Study of Income Dynamics*. Retrieved October 3, 2002, from http://www.isr.umich.edu/src/psid/overview.html

2. Martin, J., Curtin, S., Saulnier, M., & Mousavi, J. (1998). *The Matched Multiple Birth file* (Data set overview). [Electronic version]. Hyattsville, MA: National Center for Health Statistics. Retrieved May 5, 2002, from ftp://ftp.cdc.gov/pub/Health_Statistics/NCHS/datasets/mmb/

3. National Center for Health Statistics. (n.d). Table 1. Number of matched, unmatched, and incomplete records of twins and triplets by perinatal outcome: United States, 1995–1997. [Electronic version]. Hyattsville, MA: National Center for Health Statistics. Retrieved May 5, 2002, from ftp://ftp.cdc.gov/pub/Health_Statistics/NCHS/datasets/mmb/

4. Odds of having twins and higher.

5. In some cases father's birth weight status was unavailable. Such missing data could mean that, in the analyses that follow, income effects would not be adequately controlled for. However, even when dropping all cases that lacked parental birth weight data, we saw no change in our results. This lack of a difference was probably because cases missing data on father's birth weight were more likely to have lower socioeconomic statuses.

6. Gross, R., Spiker, D., & Haynes, C. (Eds.). (1997).

7. Bennett, F. (1997).

8. Smith, T., Young, B., Bae, Y., Choy, S., & Alsalam, N. (1997); National Center for Educational Statistics, (2001, March). See also Hacker, A. (2001, April 11).

9. Grossman, S., Handlesman, Y., & Davies, A. (1974). Birth weight in Israel, 1968–1970: Effects of birth order and maternal origin. *Journal of Biosocial Sciences, 6,* 43–58; Kramer, J. (1987). Intrauterine growth and gestation determinants. *Pediatrics, 80,* 502.

10. Blau, P., & Duncan. O. (1967). *The American occupational structure.* New York: John Wiley & Sons.

11. Krulewitch, C., Herman, A., Yu, K., & Johnson, Y. (1997). Does changing paternity contribute to the risk of intrauterine growth retardation? *Pediatric and Perinatal Epidemeology, 11(suppl),* 41–47.

12. Abma, J., Chandra, A., Mosher, W., Peterson, L., & Piccinino, L. (1996). *Fertility, family planning and women's health: New data from 1995 National Survey of Family Growth* (Vital Health Statistics Report no. 23[19]). Hyattsville, MA: National Center for Health Statistics.

13. Marisiglio, W., & Mott, F. (1988). Does wanting to become pregnant with a first child affect subsequent maternal behavior and infant birth weight? *Journal of Marriage and the Family, 50,* 1023–36.

14. Webb, R., & Shaw, N. (2001); Imaizumi, Y. (2001). Infant mortality rates in single, twin and triplet births, and influencing factors in Japan, 1995–1998. *Pediatric and Perinatal Epidemiology, 15,* 346–51.

15. Geronimus, A. (1996); Hardy, J., Shapiro, S., Astone, N., Miller, T., Brooks-Gunn, J., & Hilton, S. (1997).

16. Garn, S., & Petzold, A. (1981). Characteristics of the mother and child in teenage pregnancy. *American Journal of Diseases of Children, 137,* 365–68; Naeye, R. (1981).

17. Strobino, D., Ensminger, M., Young, K., & Nanda, J. (1995); Geronimus, A., & Korenman, S. (1993).

18. McLanahan, S., & Sandefur, G. (1994). *Growing up with a single parent.* Cambridge, MA: Harvard University Press; Hardy, J., Shapiro, S., Astone, N., Miller, T., Brooks-Gunn, J., & Hilton, S. (1997).

19. Geronimus, A., Korenman, S., & Hillemeir, M. (1994). Does young maternal age adversely affect child development? Evidence from cousin comparisons in the U.S. *Population and Development Review, 20,* 585–609.

20. Abel, M. (1997). Low birth weight and interactions between traditional risk factors. *Journal of Genetic Psychology, 158,* 443–56.

21. McLanahan, S. (1997). Parental absence or poverty: Which matters more? In G. Duncan, and J. Brooks-Gunn (Eds.), *Consequences of growing up poor* (pp. 35–48). New York: Russell Sage Foundation.

22. Link, B., & Phelan, J. (1995).

23. Benasich, A., & Brooks-Gunn, J. (1996). Maternal attitudes and knowledge of child-rearing: Associations with family and child outcomes. *Child Development, 67,* 1186–205.

24. Ventura, S., Martin, J., Curtin, S., Mathews, T., & Park, M. (2000); Martin, J., Hamilton, B., Ventura, S., Menacher, F., & Park, M. (2002).

25. Lieberman, E., Ryan, K., Monson, R., & Schoenbaum, S. (1987); Cooper, R. (1993). Health and the social status of blacks in the United States. *Annual Epidemiology, 3,* 137–44; Krieger, N., & Fee, E. (1994). Social class: The missing link in U.S. health data. *Journal of Health Services, 24,* 25–44.

26. Maxwell, N. (1994). For a further discussion of some of the complexities of race differences in educational attainment, see Conley, D. (1999).

27. It should be noted that we tested models with several different constructs of income—such as logged income and dummy variables—and we found no difference in our results across these various constructs. For a discussion of Orshansky ratios, see Ruggles, P. (1990). *Drawing the line: Alternative poverty measures and their implications for public policy.* Washington, DC: Urban Institute Press.

28. Such a short time period may be affected by measurement error since income tends to vary over time. However, in sibling comparisons a longer measure significantly reduces the variation in income across siblings and, therefore, may underestimate the effects of income. Neither of these problems should be a very large concern, though, since models with a longer measure of income did not yield significantly different results than those reported here.

29. Duncan, G., & Brooks-Gunn, J. (1997). Income effects across the lifespan: Integration and interpretation. In G. Duncan & J. Brooks-Gunn (Eds.), *Consequences of growing up poor* (pp. 596–611). New York: Russell Sage Foundation; Duncan, G., Brooks-Gunn, J., Yeung, W., & Smith, J. (1998).

30. Collins, J., & Shay, D. (1994).

31. Rogers, I., Emmett, P., Baker, D., & Golding, J. (1998); Avruch, S., & Cackley, A. (1995).

32. Gortmaker, S. (1979); English, P., Paul, B., Eskenazi, B., & Christianson, R. (1994).

33. For a review, see Aber, J., Bennett, N., Conley, D., & Li, J. (1997).

34. Bradley, R., Whiteside, L., Mundfrom, D., Casey, P., Kehheher, K., & Pope, S. (1994); Elder, G., Van Nguyen, T., & Caspi, A. (1995).

35. Cameron, S., & Heckman, J. (1993).

36. Cameron, S., & Heckman, J. (1993).

37. Horn, L., & Carroll, C. (1996).

38. Panel Study of Income Dynamics. (1995). *Interview year, computer assisted interview documentation* (Section M: Education). Retrieved August 15, 2002, from http://www.isr.umisch.edu/src/psid/cai_doc/1995_Interview_Year /1995_Interview_Year.htm

39. Panel Study of Income Dynamics. (1995).

40. Panel Study of Income Dynamics. (1995).

41. Hoyert, D., Arias, E., Smith, B., Murphy, S., & Kochanek, K. (2001).

42. Anderson, R. (2001). Deaths: Leadings causes for 1999. *National Vital Statistics Report, 49(11)*. Hyattsville, MA: National Center for Health Statistics.

43. For examples of this "first difference" method in very different contexts, see, for example, Duncan, G., Yeung, J., Brooks-Gunn, J., & Smith, J. (1998). How much does childhood poverty affect the life chances of children? *American Sociological Review, 63,* 406–23; Firebaugh, G., & Beck, F. (1994). Does economic growth benefit the masses? Growth, dependence, and welfare in the Third World." *American Sociological Review, 59,* 631–53.

Bibliography

Abel, M. (1997). Low birth weight and interactions between traditional risk factors. *Journal of Genetic Psychology, 158,* 443–56.

Aber, J., Bennett, N., Conley, D., & Li, J. (1997). The effects of poverty on child health and development. *Annual Review of Public Health, 18,* 463–83.

Abma, J., Chandra, A., Mosher, W., Peterson, L., & Piccinino, L. (1996). *Fertility, family planning and women's health: New data from 1995 National Survey of Family Growth* (Vital Health Statistics Report no. 23 [19]). Hyattsville, MA: National Center for Health Statistics.

Adairs, L., & Popkin, B. (1996). Low birth weight reduces the likelihood of breast-feeding among Filipino infants. *Journal of Nutrition, 126,* 103–12.

Adler, N., Boyce, T., & Chesney, M. (1994). SES and health: The challenge of the gradient. *American Psychologist, 49,* 15–24.

Administration for Children and Families. (2002). Fact Sheets: Welfare: Temporary Assistance for Needy Families. Retrieved August 15, 2002, from http://www.acf.dhhs.gov/news/facts/tanf.html

Alderman, B., Baron, A., & Salvitz, D. (1987). Maternal exposure to neighborhood carbon monoxide and risk of low infant birth weight. *Public Health Report, 102,* 410–14.

Alexander, G., Tompkins, M., Altekruse, J., & Hornung, C. (1985). Racial differences in the relation of birth weight and gestational age to neonatal mortality. *Public Health Reports, 100(5),* 539–47.

Amante, A., Borgiani, P., Gimelfarb, A., & Gloria-Bottini, F. (1996). Interethnic variability in birth weight and genetic background: A study of placental alkaline phosphates. *American Journal of Physical Anthropology, 1010,* 449–53.

Anderson, P. (1972). More is different: Broken symmetry and the nature of the hierarchical structure of science. *Science, 177(4047)*, 393–96.

Anderson, R. (2001). Deaths: Leadings causes for 1999. *National Vital Statistics Report, 49(11)*. Hyattsville, MA: National Center for Health Statistics.

Antonov, A. (1947). Children born during the siege of Leningrad in 1947. *Journal of Pediatrics, 30*, 250.

Averett, S., & Korenman, S. (1996). The economic reality of the beauty myth. *Journal of Human Resources, 31*, 304–30.

Avruch, S., & Cackley, A. (1995). Savings achieved by giving WIC benefits to women prenatally. *Public Health Reports, 110*, 27–34.

Bader, D., Kamos, A., Lwe, C., Platzker, A., Stabile, M., & Keens, T. (1987). Childhood sequelae of infant lung disease: Exercise and pulmonary function abnormalities after bronchoulmonary dysplasia. *Journal of Pediatrics, 110*, 693–99.

Baird, P. (1994). The role of genetics in population health. In R. Evans, M. Barer, & T. Marmot (Eds.), *Why are some people healthy and others not?* (pp. 133–60). New York: Aldine De Gruyter.

Bakketeig, L., Jacobsen, G., Hoffman, H., Lindmark, G., Bergsjo, P., & Molne, K. (1993). Pre-pregnancy risk factors of small-for-gestational-age births among parous women in Scandinavia. *Acta Obstetrica Gynecologica Scandinavia, 72*, 273–79.

Behrman, J., & Rosenzweig, M. (2001). *The returns to increasing body weight* (Working Paper No. 01-052). Phildelphia: University of Pennsylvania, Pennsylvania Institute for Economic Research.

Benasich, A., & Brooks-Gunn, J. (1996). Maternal attitudes and knowledge of child-rearing: Associations with family and child outcomes. *Child Development, 67*, 1186–205.

Benefits of breastfeeding could last for years. (1998, January 9). *The Toronto Star*, p. D2.

Bennett, F. (1988). Neurodevelopmental outcomes in low birthweight infants: The role of developmental intervention. In R. Guthrie (Ed.), *Neonatal intensive care: Clinics in critical care medicine* (pp. 221–50). New York: Churchill Livingstone.

Bennett, F. (1997). The LBW, premature infant. In R. Gross, D. Spiker, & C. Haynes (Eds.), *Helping low birth weight, premature babies: The infant health and development program* (pp. 3–16). Stanford, CA: Stanford University Press.

Bennett, F. (1998). Neurodevelopmental outcomes in low birth weight infants: The role of developmental intervention. In R. Guthrie (Ed.), *Neonatal intensive care: Clinics in critic care medicine* (pp. 121–250). New York: Churchill Livingstone.

Bennett, N. (1983). *Sex selection of children*. New York: Academic Press.

Binsacca, D., Ellis, J., Martin, D., & Petitti, D. (1987). Factors associated with low birthweight in an inner-city population: The role of financial problems. *American Journal of Public Health, 77*, 505–6.

Blakemore, B. (2000, July 5). An ethical dilemma. Retrieved July 15, 2000, from http://www.abcnews.com

Blau, P., & Duncan, O. (1967). *The American occupational structure*. New York: John Wiley & Sons.

Bloom, B. (1964). *Stability and change in human characteristics*. New York: John Wiley & Sons.

Borjas, G. (1990). Immigration and self selection. In R. Freeman & R. Aboard (Eds.), *Immigration, trade and the labor market* (pp. 29–76). Chicago, IL: University of Chicago Press.

Bradley, R., Whiteside, L., Mundform, D., Casey, P., Kehheher, K., & Pope, S. (1994). Early indications of resilience and their relation to experiences in the home environments of low birth weight, premature children living in poverty. *Child Development, 65,* 346–60.

Breast-fed babies' IQs higher, study says. (1999, September 23). *The Gazette,* p. B1.

Breslow, N., PelDotto, J., Brown, G., Kumar, S., Ezhuthachan, K., Hunfnagle, K., et al. (1994). A gradient relationship between low birth weight and IQ at age 6 years. *Archives of Pediatric and Adolescent Medicine, 148,* 377–83.

Brooks, A., Johnson, P., Pawson, M., & Abdalla, H. (1995). Birth weight: Nature or nurture? *Early Human Development, 42,* 29–35.

Brooks-Gunn, J., Duncan, G., & Maritato, N. (1997). Poor families, poor outcomes: The well-being of children. In G. Duncan & J. Brooks-Gunn (Eds.), *Consequences of growing up poor* (pp. 1–17). New York: Russell Sage Foundation.

Brooks-Gunn, J., Gross, R., Kraemer, H., Spiker, D., & Shapiro, S. (1992). Enhancing the cognitive outcomes of low birth weight, premature infants: For whom is intervention most effective? *Pediatrics, 89,* 1209–15.

Brooks-Gunn, J., Klebanov, P., & Duncan, G. (1996). Ethnic differences in children's intelligence test scores: Role of economic deprivation, home environment and maternal characteristics. *Child Development, 67,* 396–408.

Brown, L., Renner, M., & Flavin, C. (1997). *Vital signs*. New York: W. W. Norton.

Buescher, P., Larson, L., & Lenihan, A. (1993). Prenatal WIC participation can reduce low birth weight and newborn medical costs: A cost benefit analysis of WIC participation in North Carolina. *Journal of the American Dietetic Association, 93,* 163–66.

Bugental, D., Blue, J., & Jeffrey, L. (1990). Caregiver beliefs and dysphoric affect directed to difficult children. *Developmental Psychology, 26,* 631–38.

Bureau of Labor Statistics. (2002). Table 10: Employed persons by occupation, race, and sex. Retrieved February 7, 2002, from www.bls.gov/cps

Byrd, R., & Weitzman, M. (1994). Predictors of early grade retention among children in the United States. *Pediatrics, 93,* 481–87.

Cameron, S., & Heckman, J. (1993). The nonequivalence of high school equivalents. *Journal of Labor Economics, 11,* 1–47.

Cassel, J. (1976). The contribution of the social environment to host resistance. *American Journal of Epidemiology, 104,* 107–23.

Catalano, R., & Hartig, T. (2001). Communal bereavement and the incidence of very low birth weight in Sweden. *Journal of Health and Social Behavior, 42,* 333–41.

Catalano, R. (1991). The health effects of economic insecurity. *American Journal of Public Health, 81,* 1148–58.

Catalano, R., & Sexner, S. (1992). The effect of ambient threats to employment on low birth weight. *Journal of Health and Social Behavior, 33,* 363–77.

Centers for Disease Control, National Center for Environmental Health. (n.d.). Asthma control programs and activities related to children and adolescents: Reducing costs and improving quality of life. Retrieved January 12, 2002, from http://www.cdc.gov/nceh/airpollution/asthma/children.htm

Centers for Disease Control, National Center for Environmental Health. (2001, December 22). Blood lead levels in young children: United States and selected states, 1996–1999. *Morbidity and Mortality Weekly Report, 49(50),* 1133–37. [Electronic Version]. Retrieved January 12, 2002, from http://www.cdc.gov/mmwr/preview/mmwrhtml/mm4950a3.htm

Centers for Disease Control, National Center for Environmental Health. (n.d.). CDC's lead poisoning prevention program. Retrieved January 12, 2002, from http://www.cdc.gov/nceh/lead/lead.htm

Centers for Disease Control, National Center for Health Statistics. (1993). *Health, United States, 1992.* Hyattsville, MD: Author.

Centers for Disease Control, National Center for Health Statistics. (1998). Tables from the Linked Birth/Infant Death File. Retrieved May 16, 2000, from http://www.cdc.gov/nchswww/datawh/statab/unpubd/mortabs.htm

Centers for Disease Control, National Center for Health Statistics. (1999, September 14). Multiple birth rate for older women is sky rocketing (news release). Retrieved May 5, 2002, from http://www.cdc.gov/nchs/releases/99facts/multiple.htm

Centers for Disease Control, National Center for Health Statistics. (n.d.). Table 1. Number of matched, unmatched, and incomplete records of twins and triplets by perinatal outcome: United States, 1995–1997. [Electronic version]. Hyattsville, MA: National Center for Health Statistics. Retrieved May 5, 2002, from ftp://ftp.cdc.gov/pub/Health_Statistics/NCHS/datasets/mmb/

Cervantes, A., Keith, L., & Wyshak, G. (1999). Adverse birth outcomes among native-born and immigrant women: Replicating national evidence regarding Mexicans at the local level. *Maternal and Child Health Journal, 3,* 99–109.

Charles, A. (2001, May 15). Scientists find faulty DNA clue to breast cancer. *The Independent,* p. 4.

Cheung, V., Bocking, A., & Dasilva, O. (1995). Preterm discordant twins: What birth weight is significant? *American Journal of Obstetric Gynecology, 172,* 955–59.

Chiteji, N., & Stafford, F. (2000). Asset ownership across generations. Levy Institute for Economics, Working Paper no. 314.

Cicirelli, V. (1969). *The impact of Head Start: An evaluation of the effects of Head Start on children's cognitive and affective development* (Report No. PB 184 328, presented to the Office of Economic Opportunity). Washington, DC: Westinghouse Learning Corporation.

Colie, C. (1993). Male mediated terateogenesis. *Reproductive toxicology, 7,* 3–9.

Collins, J., & David, R. (1992). Differences in neonatal mortality by race, income and prenatal care. *Ethnicity and Disease, 2,* 18–26.

Collins, J., & David, R. (1993). Race and birth weight in biracial infants. *American Journal of Public Health, 83*, 1125–29.

Collins, J., & Shay, K. (1994). Prevalence of low birth weight among Hispanic infants with United States-born and foreign-born mothers: The effect of urban poverty. *American Journal of Epidemiology, 139*, 184–92.

Collins, M., Halsey, C., & Anderson, C. (1991). Emerging development sequelae in the "normal" extremely low birth weight infant. *Pediatrics, 88*, 115–20.

Columbia University, National Center for Children in Poverty. (2001, June). Child poverty fact sheet: June 2001. Retrieved September 21, 2002, from http://cpmcnet.columbia.edu/dept/nccp/ycpfo1.html

Committee on National Statistics, Panel on Poverty and Family Assistance. (1995). *Measuring poverty: A new approach, A report from the NAS panel on poverty and family assistance: Concepts, information needs, and measurement methods.* Washington, DC: Author.

Conger, R., Conger, K., Elder, G., Lorenz, F., Simons, R., & Whitbeck, L. (1992). A family process model of economic hardship and adjustment of early adolescent boys. *Child Development, 63*, 526–41.

Conger, R., Ge, X., Elder, G., Lorenz, F., & Simons, R. (1994). Economic stress, coercive family process and developmental problems of adolescence. *Child Development, 65*, 541–61.

Conley, D. (1999). *Being black, living in the red.* Berkeley and Los Angeles: University of California Press.

Conley, D., Bennett, N., & Li, J. (1999). *Is biology destiny or destiny biology? Poverty, education, and intergenerational aspects of low birth weight.* Unpublished Manuscript.

Cooper, R. (1993). Health and the social status of blacks in the United States. *Annual Epidemiology, 3*, 137–44.

Cooper, R. (1994). A note on the biological concept of race and its application in epidemiology research. *American Heart Journal, 108*, 715–23.

Cooper, R., Goldenberg, R., Das, A., Elder, N., Swain, M., Norman, G., et al. (1996). The preterm prediction study: Maternal stress is associated with spontaneous preterm birth at less than thirty-five weeks' gestation. *American Journal of Obstetrics and Gynecology, 175*, 1286–92.

Copley, J. (1999). A runt for life. *New Scientist, 161*, 14.

Corner, B. (1960). *Prematurity: The diagnosis, care and disorders of the premature infant.* Springfield, IL.: Thomas Books.

Coughlin, T., Ku, L., & Holahan, J. (1994). *Medicaid since the 1980s: Costs, coverage, and the shifting alliance between the federal government and the states* (pp. 47–61). Washington, DC: Urban Institute Press.

Coven. M. (2002, February 14). *An introduction to TANF* (Center on Budget and Policy Priorities Policy Report). [Electronic Version]. Washington, DC: Center on Budget and Policy Priorities. Retrieved March 20, 2002, from http://www.cbpp.org/1-22-02tanf2.pdf.

Crawley, R., McKwown, T., & Record, R. (1954). Paternal stature and birth weight. *American Journal of Public Health, 6*, 448–56.

Currie, J., & Thomas, D. (1995). Does Head Start make a difference? *American Economic Review, 85*, 341–64.

Daniels, C. (1997). Between fathers and fetuses: The social construction of male reproduction and the politics of fetal harm. *Signs, 22,* 579–616.

Danziger, S. (2000). *Approaching the limit: Early national lessons from welfare reform* (working paper). Ann Arbor, MI: University of Michigan, Poverty Research and Training Center.

Davey-Smith, G., Shipley, M., & Rose, G. (1990). Magnitude and causes of socioeconomic differentials in mortality: Further evidence from the White-hall study. *Journal of Epidemiology and Community Health, 44,* 265–70.

David, R., & Collins, J. (1997). Differing birth weight among infants of U.S.-born blacks, African-born blacks and U.S.-born whites. *New England Journal of Medicine, 337,* 1209–14.

Davis, D. (1991). Paternal smoking and fetal health. *Lancet, 337,* 123.

Denton, M., & Walters, V. (1999). Gender differences in structure and behavioral determinants of health: An analysis of the social production of health. *Social Science and Medicine, 48,* 1221–35.

Department of Health and Social Security. (1970). *Confidential inquiry into post-neonatal deaths, 1964–1966* (Reports on Public Medical Subjects No. 125). London: Her Majesty's Stationery Office.

DES Action. Health risks and care for DES daughters. Retrieved January 12, 2002, from http://www.desaction.org

Dobson, B. (1994). A WIC primer. *Journal of Human Lactation, 10,* 199–202.

Dressler, W. (1993). Health in the African American community: Accounting for health inequalities. *Medical Anthropology Quarterly, 7,* 320–45.

Dubay, L. (2002). Children's eligibility for Medicaid and SCHIP: A view from 2002 (New Federalism: National Survey of America's Families Series, Policy Review Paper No. B-41 in Series). [Electronic version]. Washington, DC: Urban Institute Press. Retrieved March 20, 2002, from http://www.urban.org

Duncan, G., & Brooks-Gunn, J. (1997). Income effects across the life span: integration and interpretation. In G. Duncan & J. Brooks-Gunn (Eds.), *Consequences of growing up poor* (pp. 596–610). New York: Russell Sage Foundation.

Duncan, G., & Brooks-Gunn, J. (Eds). (1997). *Consequences of growing up poor.* New York: Russell Sage Foundation.

Duncan, G., & Laren, D. (1990, February 13). *Neighborhood and family correlates of low birth weight: Preliminary results on births to black women from the PSID-geocode file* (research report). Ann Arbor: University of Michigan, Survey Research Center.

Duncan, G., & Rodgers, W. (1988). Has children's poverty become more persistent? *American Sociological Review, 56,* 361–75.

Duncan, G., Yeung, J., Brooks-Gunn, J., Smith, J. (1998). How Much Does Childhood Poverty Affect the Life Chances of Children? *American Sociological Review, 63,* 406–23.

Duncan, G., & Brooks-Gunn, J. (1997). Income effects across the life-span: Integration and interpretation. In G. Duncan & J. Brooks-Gunn (Eds.), *Consequences of growing up poor* (pp. 596–611). New York: Russell Sage Foundation.

Dunn, H., Crichton, R., Grunau, A., McBurney, A., McCormmick, A., Roberston, A., et al. (1980). Neurological, psychological and educational sequelae of low birth weight. *Brain Development, 2,* 57–67.

Duster, T. (1990). *Back door to eugenics.* New York: Routledge.

Easterlin, R. (1980). *Birth and fortune: The impact of numbers on personal welfare.* New York: Basic Books.

Elder, G., Van Nguyen, T., & Caspi, A. (1995). Linking family hardship to children's lives. *Child Development, 56,* 361–75.

Ellen, I. (2000). Is segregation bad for your health? The case of low birth weight. Brookings-Wharton Papers on Urban Affairs. (Pp. 203–29).

Elwood, C., & Hoem, J. (1999). Low-weight neonatal survival paradox in the Czech Republic. *American Journal of Epidemiology, 149,* 447–53.

Engles, F. (1967). *The process of capitalist production* (S. Moore & E. Aveling, Eds & Trans.). New York: International Publishers. (Original work published 1867).

English, P., Paul, B., Eskenazi, B., & Christianson, R. (1994). Black-white differences in serum cotinine levels among pregnant women and subsequent effects on infant birth weight. *American Journal of Public Health, 84,* 1439–43.

Epstein, H. (2001, April 12). Time of indifference. *New York Review of Books, 48(3),* 12–15.

Ernster, V. (1988). Trends in smoking, cancer risk, and cigarette promotion. *Cancer, 62,* 1702–12.

Escalona, S. (1987). *Critical issues in the early development of premature infants.* New Haven, CT: Yale University Press.

Eskenazi, B., Prehn, A., & Christianson, R. (1995). Passive and active maternal smoking as measured by serum cotinine: The effects on birth weight. *American Journal of Public Health, 85,* 395–98.

Evans, R., Barer, M., & Marmot, T. (1994). *Why are some people healthy and others are not? Determinants of health of populations.* New York: DeGruyter Press.

Festinger, L. (1957). *A theory of cognitive dissonance.* Stanford: Stanford University Press.

Firebaugh, G., & Beck, F. (1994). Does economic growth benefit the masses? Growth, dependence, and welfare in the Third World. *American Sociological Review, 59,* 631–53.

Foster, H. (1997). The enigma of low birth weight and race. *New England Journal of Medicine, 337,* 1232–33.

Freidler, H., & Wheeling, H. (1997). Behavioral effects in offspring of male mice injected with opioids prior to mating. In *Protracted effects of perinatal drug dependence, vol. 2. Pharmacology, biochemistry and behavior* (pp. s23–s28). Fayetteville, NY: ANKHO International.

Friedman, S., Jacobs, B., & Weithmann, M. (1982). Preterms of low medical risk: Spontaneous behaviors and soothability at expected date of birth. *Infant Behavioral Development, 5,* 3–10.

Frisbie, W., Cho, Y., & Hummer, R. (2001). Immigration and the health of Asian and American Pacific Islander adults in the U.S. *American Journal of Epidemiology, 153,* 372–80.

Frisbie, W., Forbes, D., & Pullman, S. (1996). Compromised birth outcomes and infant mortality among racial and ethnic groups. *Demography, 33,* 469–81.

Friscella, K., & Franks, P. (1997). Poverty or income inequality as a predictor of mortality: Longitudinal cohort study. *British Medical Journal, 314,* 1724–28.

Garn, S., & Petzold, A. (1981). Characteristics of the mother and child in teenage pregnancy. *American Journal of Diseases of Children, 137,* 365–68.

Gene may affect anxiety disorder. (2001, April 32). *San Diego Union-Tribune,* p. A11.

Gene may predispose some boxers to brain trauma, study finds. (1997, July 9). *Star Tribune,* p. 9A.

Geronimus, A. (1996). Black/white differences in the relationship of maternal age to birthweight: A population-based test of the weathering hypothesis. *Social Science and Medicine, 42,* 589–97.

Geronimus, A. (1997). Teenage childbearing and personal responsibility: An alternative view. *Political Science Quarterly, 112,* 405–30.

Geronimus, A., Bound, J., Waidmann, T., Hillereier, M., & Burns, P. (1996). Excess mortality among blacks and whites in the United States. *New England Journal of Medicine, 335,* 1552–58.

Geronimus, A., & Korenman, S. (1993). Maternal youth or family background? On the health disadvantages of infants with teenage mothers. *American Journal of Epidemiology, 137,* 213–25.

Geronimus, A., Korenman, S., & Hillemeir, M. (1994). Does young maternal age adversely affect child development? Evidence from cousin comparisons in the U.S. *Population and Development Review, 20,* 585–609.

Gertz, L., Dobson, V., & Luna, B. (1994). Development of grating acuity, letter acuity and visual fields in small-for-gestational-age preterm infants. *Early Human Development, 40,* 59–71.

Goldblatt, P. (1990). *Longitudinal study: Mortality and social organization.* London: Her Majesty's Stationery Office.

Goodman, R., & Moltulsky, A. (1984). Genetic diseases among Ashkenazi Jews. *Mankind Quarterly, 25,* 169–79.

Gortmaker, S. (1979). Poverty and infant mortality in the United States. *American Sociological Review, 44,* 280–97.

Gould, J., & LeRoy, S. (1998). Socioeconomic status and low birth weight: A racial comparison. *Pediatrics, 82,* 896–904.

Gould, J., Davey, B., & LeRoy, S. (1989). Socioeconomic differentials and neonatal mortality: Racial comparison of California singletons. *Pediatrics, 83,* 181–86.

Gravelle, H. (1998). How much of the relationship between population mortality and unequal distribution of income is a statistical artifact. *British Medical Journal, 316,* 382–85.

Gross, R. (1997). The primary child outcomes. In R. Gross, D. Spiker, & C. Haynes (Eds.), *Helping low birth weight, premature babies: The Infant Health and Development Program* (pp. 139–54). Stanford, CA: Stanford University Press.

Gross, R., Spiker, D., & Haynes, C. (Eds.). (1997). *Helping low birth weight, premature babies: The infant health and development program.* Stanford, CA: Stanford University Press.

Grossman, S., Handlesman, Y., & Davies, A. (1974). Birth weight in Israel, 1968–1970: Effects of birth order and maternal origin. *Journal of Biosocial Sciences, 6,* 43–58.

Guendelman, S., Gould, J., Hudes, M., & Eskenazi, B. (1990). Generational differences in perinatal health among the Mexican American population: Findings from HANES. *American Journal of Public Health, 80,* 61–65.

Gundersen, C., LeBlanc, M., & Kuhn, B. (1999). *The changing food assistance landscape: The Food Stamp program in a post-welfare reform environment* (Agricultural Economics Report No. 773). Washington, DC: U.S. Department of Agriculture, Economics Research Service).

Hack, M., Flannery, D., Schluchter, M., Cartar, L., Borawski, E., & Klein, N. (2002). Outcomes in young adulthood for very low birth weight infants. *New England Journal of Medicine, 346,* 149–57.

Hack, M., Klein, N., & Flannery, D. (2002). Correspondence: Outcomes in young adulthood for very-low-birth-weight infants: The authors reply. *New England Journal of Medicine, 347,* 142.

Hacker, A. (2001, April 11). How are women doing? *New York Review of Books, 49(6),* 63–66.

Hagberg, B., Hagberg, G., Olow, I., & Von Wendt, L. (1989). The changing panorama of cerebral palsy in Sweden: The birth year period 1979–1982. *Acta Pediatrica Scandinavia, 78,* 283–90.

Haines, M., Craig, L., & Weiss, T. (2000). *Development, health, nutrition, and mortality: the Case of the 'antebellum puzzle' in the United States* (Historical Paper 130). Cambridge, MA: National Bureau of Economic Research.

Hanson, T., McLanahan, S., & Thomson, E. (1997). Economic resources, parent practices, and children's well-being. In G. Duncan & J. Brooks-Gunn (Eds.), *Consequences of growing up poor* (pp. 190–238). New York: Russell Sage Foundation.

Hardy, J., Shapiro, S., Astone, N., Miller, T., Brooks-Gunn, J., & Hilton, S. (1997). Adolescent childbearing revisited: The age of inner-city mothers at delivery is a determinant of their children's self-sufficiency at age 27 to 33. *Pediatrics, 100,* 802–9.

Health Care Financing Administration. (2000). Medicaid eligibility. Retrieved August 15, 2001, from http://www.hcfa.gov/medicaid/medicaid.htm

Health Care Financing Administration. (2002). Special Medicaid coverage for pregnant women. Retrieved March 11, 2002, from http://www.hcfa.gov/hiv/subpg4.htm

Hedegaard, M., Henriksen, T., Secher, N., Hack, M., & Sabroe, S. (1996). Do stressful life events affect duration of gestation and risk of preterm delivery? *Epidemiology, 7,* 339–45.

Hensley, S. (2001, May 15). Gene linked to breast cancer yields secrets. *Wall Street Journal,* p. B16.

Herrnstein, R., & Murray, C. (1996). *The bell curve: Intelligence and class struggle in American life.* New York: Free Press.

Hill, M. (1992). *The panel study of income dynamics: A user's guide*. Newbury Park, CA: Sage.

Himmelmann, A., Svensson, A., & Handsson, L. (1994). Relation of maternal blood pressure during pregnancy to birth weight and blood pressure in children: The Hypertension Study. *Journal of Internal Medicine, 235*, 347–52.

Hobel, C., Dunkel-Schetter, C., Roesch, S., Castro, L., & Arora, C. (1999). Maternal plasma corticotropin-releasing hormone associated with stress at 20 weeks' gestation in pregnancies ending in preterm delivery. *American Journal of Obstetrics and Gynecology, 180*, 257–64.

Holahan, J. (1997). *Expanding insurance coverage for children* (Policy Report). [Electronic version]. Washington, DC: The Urban Institute. Retrieved March 20, 2002, from http://www.urban.org

Holden, C. (1990). Head Start enters adulthood. *Science, 247*, 1400.

Hollier, L., McIntire, D., & Leveno, K. (1999). Outcome of twin pregnancies according to interpair birth weight differences. *Obstetrics and Gynecology, 94(6)*, 1006–10.

Horn, L., & Carroll, C. (1996). *Nontraditional undergraduates: Trends in enrollment from 1986 to 1992 and persistence and attainment among 1989–90 beginning post-secondary students* (Statistical Analysis Report No. 97578). Washington, DC: National Center for Education Statistics.

House, J., Kessler, R., Herzog, A., Mero, R., Kinner, A., & Breslow, M. (1990). Age, socioeconomic status and health. *Milbank Quarterly, 68*, 383–411.

Howes, C., & Olenick, M. (1986). Family and child influences on toddlers' compliance. *Child Development, 26*, 292–303.

Howes, C., & Stewart, P. (1987). Child's play with adults, toys, and peers: An examination of family and child care influences. *Developmental Psychology, 23*, 423–30.

Hoyert, D., Arias, E., Smith, B., Murphy, S., & Kochanek, K. (2001). Deaths: Final data for 1999. *National Vital Statistics Reports, 49(8)*. Hyattsville, MA: National Center for Health Statistics.

Hummer, R. (1993). Racial differences in infant mortality in the U.S.: An examination of social and health determinants. *Social Forces, 72*, 529–54.

Hummer, R. (1996). Black-white differences in health and mortality: A review and conceptual model. *Sociological Quarterly, 37*, 108.

Hunt, J. (1961). *Intelligence and experience*. New York: Ronald Press.

Illsley, R. (1955). Social class selection and class differences in relation to still-births and infant death. *British Medical Journal, 2*, 1520–24.

Illsley, R., & Mulley, K. (1985). The health needs of disadvantaged client groups. In W. Holland, R. Detels, & G. Knox (Eds.), *Oxford textbook of public health*. (pp. 389–402). Oxford, UK: Oxford University Press.

Imaizumi, Y. (2001). Infant mortality rates in single, twin and triplet births, and influencing factors in Japan, 1995–1998. *Pediatric and Perinatal Epidemiology, 15*, 346–51.

Institute for Social Research, University of Michigan. (2000, August). *An overview of the Panel Study of Income Dynamics*. Retrieved October 3, 2002, from http://www.isr.umich.edu/src/psid/overview.html

Internal Revenue Service. (2002). Child Tax Credit: Topic 606. Retrieved October 5, 2002, from www.irs.gov/tax_edu/teletax/tc606.html

Internal Revenue Service. (2002). EITC overview. Retrieved October 5, 2002, from www.irs.gov/ind_info/eitc-ovrvw.html

James, S. (1993). Racial and ethnic differences in mortality and low birth weight. *Annual Epidemiology, 3,* 130–36.

James, S. (1994). John Henryism and the health of African Americans. *Culture, Medicine and Psychiatry, 18,* 163–82.

Jencks, C., Smith, M., Acland, H., Bane, J., Cohen, D., Gintis, H., et al. (1973). *Inequality: A reassessment of the effects of family and schooling in America.* New York: Basic Books.

Judge, K. (1995). Income distribution and life expectancy. *British Medical Journal, 311,* 1282–85.

Kagamimori, S., Iibuchi, Y., & Fox, A. (1983). A comparison of socioeconomic differences in mortality between Japan, England, and Wales. *World Health Statistics Quarterly, 36,* 119–28.

Kallan, J. (1993). Race, intervening variables, and two components of low birth weight. *Demography, 30,* 489–506.

Kaplan, G. (1985). Twenty years of health in Alameda County: The Human Population Laboratory Analysis. Paper presented at the annual meeting of Society for Prospective Medicine, San Francisco.

Kennedy, B., Kawachi, I., & Prothrwo-Stith, D. (1996). Income distribution and mortality: Cross-sectional ecological study of the Robin Hood Index in the United States. *British Medical Journal, 312,* 1004–7.

Kennedy, B., Kwachi, I., Glass, I., & Prothrwo-Stith, D. (1998). Income distribution, socioeconomic status, and self-rated health: A U.S. multi-level analysis. *British Medical Journal, 317,* 917–21.

Kitagawa, E., & Hauser, P. (1973). *Differential mortality in the United States: A study in socioeconomic epidemiology.* Cambridge, MA: Harvard University Press.

Klag, M., Whelton, D., Coresh, J., Grim, C., & Kuller, L. (1991). The association of skin color with blood pressure in U.S. blacks with low socioeconomic status. *Journal of the American Medical Association, 265,* 599–602.

Klebanov, P. (1994). Classroom behavior of very low birth weight elementary school children. *Pediatrics, 94,* 700–8.

Korenman, S., & Miller, J. (1997). Effects of long-term poverty on physical health of children in the National Longitudinal Study of Youth. In G. Duncan & J. Brooks-Gunn (Eds.), *Consequences of growing up poor* (pp. 70–99). New York: Russell Sage Foundation.

Koskenvuo, M., Kaprio, J., Kesaniemi, A., & Sarna, S. (1978). Differences in mortality from ischemic heart disease by marital status and social class. *Journal of Chronic Disease, 33,* 95–106.

Kotlikoff, L., & Summers, L. (1981). The role of intergenerational transfers in aggregate capital accumulation. *Journal of Political Economy, 89,* 706–32.

Kramer, J. (1987). Intrauterine growth and gestation determinants. *Pediatrics, 80,* 502.

Kramer, M., Platt, R., Yang, H., McNamara, H., & Usher, R. (1999). Are all growth-restricted newborns created equal(ly)? *Pediatrics, 103,* 599–602.

Kreiger, N. (1990). Racial and gender discrimination: Risk factors for high blood pressure? *Social Science and Medicine, 30,* 1273–81.

Krieger, N., & Fee, E. (1994). Social class: The missing link in U.S. health data. *Journal of Health Services, 24,* 25–44.

Krukewitch, C., Herman, A., Yu, K., & Johnson, Y. (1997). Does changing paternity contribute to the risk of intrauterine growth retardation? *Pediatric and Perinatal Epidemiology, 11(suppl),* 41–47.

Ku, L., Ullman, F., & Almeida, R. (1999). *What counts? Determining Medicaid and CHIP eligibility for children.* (Urban Institute Discussion Paper No. 99-05). Washington, DC: Urban Institute Press.

Landale, N., Oropesa, R., & Gorman, B. (2000). Migration and infant death: Assimilation or selective migration among Puerto Ricans? *American Sociological Review, 65,* 888–909.

Lang, J., Lieberman, E., & Cohen, A. (1996). A comparison of risk factors for preterm labor and term small-for-gestational age birth. *Epidemiology, 7,* 369–76.

Lantz, P., House, J., Lepkowski, J., Williams, D., Mero, R., & Chen, J. (1998, August 21–25). *Socioeconomic status, health behaviors, and mortality: Results from a nationally representative prospective study of U.S. adults.* Paper presented at the American Sociological Association Annual Meeting, San Francisco.

Last, J. (Ed.). (1986). *Hypertension in public health and preventative medicine* (12th ed.). Norwalk, CT: Appelton-Century-Crofts.

LaVeist, T. (1990, Winter). Simulating the effects of poverty on the race disparity in post-neonatal mortality. *Journal of Public Health Policy, 11,* 462–73.

LaVeist, T. (1992). The political empowerment and health status of African Americans: Mapping a new territory. *American Journal of Sociology, 97,* 1080–95.

LaVeist, T. (1993). Segregation, poverty and empowerment: Health consequences for African Americans. *Milbank Quarterly, 71,* 41–64.

LeClerc, A., Lert, F., & Goldberg, M. (1984). Les inegalites sociales devant la mort en Grande Bretagne et en France. *Social Science and Medicine, 19,* 479–87.

LeClere, F., Richard, R., & Peters, K. (1997). Ethnicity and mortality in the United States: Individual and neighborhood level correlates. *Social Forces, 76,* 169–98.

Lederman, S., & Paxton, A. (1998). Maternal reporting of prepregnancy weight and birth outcome: Consistency and completeness compared with the clinical record. *Maternal and Child Health Journal, 2,* 123–26.

Leonard, C., Clyman, R., Piecuch, R., Piecuch, R., Juster, R., & Ballard, R. (1990). Effect of medical and social risk factors on outcome of prematurity and very low birth weight. *Journal of Pediatrics, 116,* 620–26.

Lewontin, R. (2000). *The triple helix: Gene, organism and environment.* Cambridge, MA: Harvard University Press.

Lieberman, E., Gremy, I., & Lang, J. (1994). Low birthweight and the timing of fetal exposure to maternal smoking. *American Journal of Public Health, 94,* 1127–31.

Lieberman, E., Ryan, K., Monson, R., & Schoenbaum, S. (1987). Risk factors accounting for racial differences in the rate of premature birth. *New England Journal of Medicine, 317,* 743–48.

Link, B., & Phelan, J. (1995). Social conditions as fundamental causes of disease. *Journal of Health and Social Behavior (Extra issue),* 80–94.

Link, B., Northridge, M., Phelan, J., & Ganz, M. (1998). Social epidemiology and the fundamental causes concept: On the structuring of effective cancer screens by socioeconomic status. *Milbank Quarterly, 76,* 375–402.

Liska, D., Brennan, N., & Bruen, B. (2001). *State level databook on health care access and financing* (3rd ed.). Washington, DC: Urban Institute Press.

Lochner, K. (1999). State inequality and individual mortality risk: A prospective multi-level study. Unpublished doctoral dissertation, Harvard University, Cambridge, MA.

Lockwood, C. (1999). Stress-associated preterm delivery: The role of corticotropin-releasing hormone. *American Journal of Obstetrics and Gynecology, 180,* 264–66.

Long, S., Kurka, R., Waters, S., & Kirby, G. (1998). *Child care assistance under welfare reform: Early responses by the states* (Assessing the New Federalism Series, Paper No. 15). [Electronic Version]. Washington, DC: Urban Institute Press. Retrieved September 27, 2002, from http://www.urban.org/Template.cfm?NavMenuID=24

Loprest, P. (1997). *Supplemental security income for children with disabilities* (Issues and Options for States Series, Paper No. A-10). [Electronic version]. Washington, DC: The Urban Institute. Retrieved March 15, 2002, http://www.urban.org/Template.cfm?NavMenuID=24

Luke, B., Williams, C., Minogue, J., & Keith, L. (1993). The changing pattern of infant mortality in the United States: The role of prenatal factors and their obstetrical implications. *Internal Journal of Gynecological Obstetrics, 40,* 199–212.

Lumey, L., & Stein, A. (1997). In-utero exposure to famine and subsequent fertility: The Dutch Famine birth cohort study. *American Journal of Public Health, 87,* 1962–66.

Lumey, L., & Van Poppel, F. (1994). The Dutch Famine of 1944–1945: Mortality and morbidity in past and present generations. *Social Historical Medicine, 7,* 229–46.

Lynge, E. (1984). Socioeconomic and occupational morality differentials in Europe. *Sozial-un Praventivmedizin, 29,* 265–67.

Mackenback, J. (1992). Socio-economic health differences in the Netherlands: A review of recent empirical findings. *Social Science and Medicine, 34,* 213–26.

Mangold, W., & Powell-Griner, E. (1991). Race of parents and infant birthweight in the United States. *Social Biology, 38,* 13–27.

Mare, R. (1990). Socioeconomic careers and differential morality among older men in the U.S. In J. Vallin, S. D'Souza, & A. Palloni (Eds.), *Measurement and Analysis of Mortality—New Approaches.* (pp. 362–87). Oxford, UK: Clarendon.

Mare, R. (1991). Five decades of educational assortative mating. *American Sociological Review, 56,* 15–32.

Marisiglio, W., & Mott, F. (1988). Does wanting to become pregnant with a first child affect subsequent maternal behavior and infant birth weight? *Journal of Marriage and the Family, 50,* 1023–36.

Marmot, M., & Theroll, T. (1988). Social class and cardiovascular disease: The contribution of work. *International Journal of Health Services, 18,* 659–74.

Marmot, M. (1986). Social inequalities in mortality: The social environment. In R. Wilkinson (Ed.), *Class and health: Research and longitudinal data* (pp. 21–33). London: Tavistock.

Marmot, M., Fuhrer, R., Ettner, S., Nadine, F., Bumpass, L., & Ryff, C. (1998). Contribution of psychosocial factors to socioeconomic differences in health. *Milbank Quarterly, 76,* 403–48.

Marmot, M., Rose, G., Shipley, M., & Hamilton, P. (1978). Employment grade and coronary heart disease in British civil servants. *Journal of Epidemiology and Community Health, 32,* 244–49.

Marmot, M., Smith, G., Stansgeld, S., Patek, C., North, F., Head, J., et al. (1991). Health inequalities among British civil servants: The Whitehall study. *Lancet, 337,* 1387–93.

Martin, J., & Park, M. (1999). Trends in twin and triplet births: 1980–97. *National Vital Statistics Report, 47.* Hyattsville, MA: National Center for Health Statistics.

Martin, J., Curtin, S., Saulnier, M., & Mousavi, J. (1998). *The Matched Multiple Birth file* (Dataset overview). [Electronic version]. Hyattsville, MA: National Center for Health Statistics. Retrieved May 5, 2002, from ftp://ftp.cdc.gov/pub/Health_Statistics/NCHS/datasets/mmb/

Martin, J., Hamilton, B., Ventura, S. Menacher, F., & Park, M. (2002). Births: Final data for 1999. *National Vital Statistics Reports, 50(5).* Hyattsville, MA: National Center for Health Statistics.

Martinez, F., Wright, A., Taussig, L., & the Group Health Medical Associates. (1994). The effect of paternal smoking on the birthweight of newborns whose mothers did not smoke. *American Journal of Public Health, 89,* 1489–91.

Martorell, R., & Habichit, J. P. (1986). Growth in early childhood in developing countries. In F. Faulkner & J. M. Tanner (Eds.), *Human growth: A comprehensive treatise, vol. 3* (pp. 241–62). New York: Plenum Press.

Massey, D. (1993). Latinos, poverty and the underclass: A new agenda for research. *Hispanic Journal of Behavioral Sciences, 15,* 449–75.

Maugh, T., & Springer, S. (1997, July 9). In the genes? Doctors may be able to predict if a fighter is susceptible to chronic brain damage. *Los Angeles Times,* p. 1.

Maxwell, N. (1994). The effects of black-white wage differences in the quality and quantity of education. *Industrial Labor Relations and Review, 47,* 249–64.

Mayer, S. (1997). *What money can't buy: Family income and children's life chances.* Cambridge, MA: Harvard University Press.

McBurney, A., & Eaves, L. (1986). Evolution of developmental and psychological test scores. In H. Dunn (Ed.), *Sequelae of low birthweight: The Vancouver Study* (pp. 54–67). Philadelphia: Lippincott.

McCormick, M., Shapiro, S., & Starfeild, B. (1980). Rehospitalization in the first year of life for high-risk survivors. *Pediatrics, 66,* 991–99.

McCormick, M., Brooks-Gunn, J., Workman-Daniels, K., & Peckham, G. (1993). Maternal rating of child health at school age: Does the Vulnerable Child Syndrome persist? *Pediatrics, 92,* 380–88.

McCormick, M., Stemmler, M., Bernbaum, J., & Farran, A. (1986), The very low birth weight transport goes home: Impact on the family. *Journal of Developmental Behavioral Pediatrics, 10,* 86–91.

McCormick, M., Workman-Daniels, K., & Brooks-Gunn, J. (1996). The behavioral and emotional well-being of school-age children with different birth weights. *Pediatrics, 97,* 18–25.

McDonal, M., Sigma, M., & Ungerer, J. (1989). Intelligence and behavioral problems in 5-year-olds in relation to representational abilities in the second year of life. *Journal of Developmental Behavioral Pediatrics, 10,* 86–91.

McGauhery, P. (1991). Social environment and vulnerability of low birth weight children: A social-epidemiological perspective. *Pediatrics, 88,* 943–53.

McKinlay, J., & McKinlay, S. (1997). Medical measures and the decline of mortality. In P. Conrad (Ed.), *The sociology of health and illness* (5th ed.). (pp. 10–23). New York: St. Martin's Press.

Mcknight, J. (1985). Health and empowerment. *Canadian Journal of Public Health, 76(suppl),* S37–S38.

McLanahan, S., & Sandefur, G. (1994). *Growing up with a single parent.* Cambridge, MA: Harvard University Press.

McLanahan, S. (1997). Parental absence or poverty: Which matters more? In G. Duncan, and J. Brooks-Gunn (Eds.), *Consequences of growing up poor* (pp. 35–48). New York: Russell Sage Foundation..

Michaelis, R., Asenbauer, C., Buchwald-Senal, M., Haas, G., & Krageboh-Mann, I. (1993). Transitory neurological findings in a population of at risk infants. *Early Human Development, 34,* 143–53.

Miller, J. (1994). Birth order, interpregnancy interval and birth outcomes among Filipino infants. *Journal of Biosocial Science, 26,* 243–59.

Modigliani, F. (1988). The role of intergenerational transfers and life cycle saving in the accumulation of wealth. *Journal of Economic Perspectives, 2,* 15–40.

Montgomery, S., Bartley, M., & Wilkinson, R. (1997). Family conflict and slow growth. *Archive of Diseases in Children, 77,* 326–30.

Montgomery, S., Bartley, M., Cook, D., & Wadsworth, M. (1996). Health and social precursors of unemployment in young men. *Journal of Epidemiology and Community Health, 50,* 415–22.

Morenoff, J. (2001). Place, race, and health: Neighborhood sources of group disparities in birthweight (PSC Research Report No. 01-482). Ann Arbor: University of Michigan, Population Studies Center.

Moron, N. (1977). Genetic aspects of prematurity. In D. Reed & F. Stanley (Eds.), *The epidemiology of prematurity* (pp. 213–30). Baltimore, MD: Urban & Schwartzenberg.

Morton, N., Chung, C., & Mi, M. (1967). *Genetics and interracial crosses in Hawaii.* Basel, Switzerland: Karger Medical & Scientific.

Moss, N., & Carver, K. (1998). The effect of WIC and Medicaid on infant mortality in the United States. *American Journal of Public Health, 88,* 1354–61.

Mosse, G. (1981). *Toward the final solution: A history of European racism.* New York: H. Fertig.

Murphy, S. (2000). Deaths: Final data for 1998. *National Vital Statistics Reports, 48(11).* Hyattsville, MA: National Center for Health Statistics.

Naeye, R. (1981). Teenaged and pre-teenaged pregnancies: Consequences of the fetal-maternal competition for nutrients. *Pediatrics, 67,* 146–50.

Nash, K., & Kramer, K. (1993). Self help for sickle cell diseases in African American communities. *Journal of Applied Behavioral Sciences, 29,* 202–15.

National Center for Children in Poverty, Research Forum on Children, Families, and the New Federalism. (2001). *Three-city findings reveal unexpected diversity among welfare leavers and stayers* (Research Report). New York: Author.

National Center for Educational Statistics. (2001, March). *Digest of Educational Statistics* (Table 248). Washington, DC: Author.

National Governors' Association. (1995, September). State Medicaid coverage of pregnant women and children. *MCH Update.* Washington, DC: Author.

National Institute of Environmental Health Services, National Toxicology Program. (n.d.). Known carcinogen: diethylstilbestrol (CAS No. 56-53-1). Research Triangle Park, NC: Author. Retrieved January 12, 2002, from http://ntpserver.niehs.nih.gov/htdocs/ARC/ARC_KC/Diethylstilbestrol.html

National Organization of Mothers of Twins Clubs, Inc. (n.d). Twinning facts. Retrieved April 20, 2002, from http://www.nomotc.org/twinning_facts.html

Navarro, V. (1990). Race or class versus race and class: Morality differentials in the United States. *Lancet, 336,* 1238–40.

Norbeck, J., DeJoseph, J., & Smith, R. (1996). A randomized trial of an empirically-driven social support intervention to prevent low birth weight among African American women. *Social Science and Medicine, 43,* 947–54.

Norton, T., Kenneth, E., Juliette, K., & Remington, P. (1988). Smoking by blacks and whites: Socioeconomic and demographic differences. *American Journal of Public Health, 78,* 1187–89.

Nystrom-Peck, M., & Lundberg, O. (1995). Short stature as an effect of economic and social conditions in childhood. *Social Science and Medicine, 41,* 733–38.

O'Campo, P., Xue, X., Wang, M., & Caughy, M. (1997). Neighborhood risk factors for low birth weight in Baltimore: A multilevel analysis. *American Journal of Public Health, 80,* 1113–19.

Odds of having twins and higher. (n.d.). Retrieved April 16, 2002, from http://www.geocities.com/factsaboutmultiples/twinbasics2.html

Ounsted, M., & Scott, A. (1982). Social class and birthweight: A new look. *Human Development, 6,* 83–89.

Overspect, M., & Moss, A. (1991). *Children's exposure to environmental cigarette smoke before and after birth* (Advanced Data Report No. 202). Hyattsville, MA: National Center for Health Statistics.

Pagan, J., & Davila, A. (1997). Obesity, occupational attainment and earnings. *Social Science Quarterly, 78,* 756–70.

Pallotto, E., Collins, J., & David, R. (2000). Enigma of maternal race and infant birth weight: A population-based study of U.S.-born black and Caribbean-born black women. *American Journal of Epidemiology, 151,* 1080–85.

Panel Study of Income Dynamics. (1995). *Interview year, computer assisted interview documentation* (Section M: Education). Retrieved August 15, 2002, from http://www.isr.umisch.edu/src/psid/cai_doc/1995_Interview_Year /1995_Interview_Year.htm

Pappas, G., Queen, S., Hadden, W., & Fisher, G. (1993). The increasing disparity between socioeconomic groups in the Untied States, 1960 to 1986. *New England Journal of Medicine, 329,* 103–15.

Parents' Place. (n.d.). Twin biology: Chorionicity of the placenta. Retrieved May 5, 2002, from http://www.parentsplace.com/pregnancy/labor/articles /0,10335,166530_111532,00.html

Parker, J., & Schoendorf, K. (1992). Influence of paternal characteristics on the risk of low birth weight. *American Journal of Public Health, 136,* 399–407.

Parker, S., Greer, S., & Zuckerman, B. (1988). Double jeopardy: The impact of poverty on early child development. *Pediatric Clinics of North America, 35(6),* 1227–40.

Partin, M., & Pallonu, A. (1995). Accounting for the recent increase in low birth weight among African Americans. *Focus, 16,* 33–37.

Pattillo-McCoy, M., & Heflin, C. (1999). Poverty in the family: Siblings of the black and white middle classes. Paper presented at the Annual Meeting of the American Sociological Association, Chicago.

Pearl, R., & Donahue, M. (1995). Four years after a pre-term birth: Children's development and their mother's beliefs and expectations. *Journal of Pediatric Psychology, 20,* 363–70.

Peterson, R. (1997, July 31). Nurturing may play a role in intelligence. *USA Today,* p. 1D.

Pevalin, D., Wade, T., Brannigan, A., & Sauve, R. (2000, August 12–16). *Adverse birth outcomes, maternal prenatal behavior and their social context.* Paper presented at the American Sociological Association Annual Meeting, Washington, DC.

Phillips, D., McCartney, K., & Scarr, S. (1987). Child care quality and children's social development. *Developmental Psychology, 23,* 537–43.

Polednak, A. (1991). Black-white differentials in infant mortality in 38 standard metropolitan statistical areas. *American Journal of Public Health, 81,* 1480–82.

Polednak, A. (1997). *Segregation, poverty and mortality in urban African Americans.* Oxford: Oxford University Press.

Polit, D., London, A., & Martinez, J. (2001. May). *The health of poor urban women: Findings from the Project on Devolution and Urban Change* (Manpower Demonstration Research Corporation Report). [Electronic Version]. New York: Manpower Demonstration Research Corporation. Retrieved October 10, 2001, from http://www.mdrc.org/Publications.htm

Pope, S., Whiteside, L., Brooks-Gunn, J., Kelleher, K., Rickert, V., Bradley, R., & Casey, P. (1993). Low-birth-weight infants born to adolescent mothers: Effects of co-residency with grandmother on child development. *Journal of the American Medical Association, 269,* 136–400.

Potter, L. (1991). Socioeconomic determinants of white and black males' life expectancy differentials, 1980. *Demography, 28,* 303–21.

Power, C., & Parsons, T. (2000). Nutritional and other influences in childhood as predictors of adult obesity. *Proceedings of the Nutrition Society, 59,* 257–72.

Power, W., & Kiely, J. (1994). The risks confronting twins: A national perspective. *American Journal of Obstetrics and Gynecology, 170,* 456–61.

Ramey, C., Bryant, D., Wasik, B., Sparling, J., Fendt, K., & Ange, L. (1992). Infant Health and Development Program for low birth weight, premature infants: Program elements, family participation, and child intelligence. *Pediatrics, 89,* 454–65.

Ramey, C., & Ramey, S. (1994). Which children benefit the most from early intervention? *Pediatrics, 94,* 1064–66.

Ramey, C., Sparling, J., Bryant, D., & Wasik, B. (1997). The intervention model. In R. Gross, D. Spiker, & C. Haynes (Eds.), *Helping low birth weight, premature babies: The Infant Health and Development Program* (pp. 17–26). Stanford, CA: Stanford University Press.

Reed, D., and Stanley, F. (Eds.). (1977). *The epidemiology of prematurity.* Baltimore, MD: Urban & Schwarzenberg.

Rich-Edwards, J. (1997). Birth weight and risk of cardiovascular disease in a cohort of women followed-up since 1976. *British Medical Journal, 35,* 396–400.

Riese, M. (1995). Neonatal temperament in full-term twin pairs discordant for birth weight. *Journal of Development and Behavioral Pediatrics, 15,* 342–47.

Riese, M. (1996). Temperamental development to 30 months of age in discordant twin pairs. *Acta geneticae medicae et gemellologiae, 45,* 439–47.

Rissahen, A. (1996). The economic and psychological consequences of obesity. *Origins and Consequences of Obesity, 201,* 194–96.

Roberston, C., Hrynchyshyn, G., Etches, P., & Pain, K. (1992). Population-based study of the incidence, complexity and severity of neurological disability among survivors weighing 500 through 1250 grams at birth: A comparison of two birth cohorts. *Pediatrics, 990,* 750–55.

Roberts, E. (1997). Neighborhood social environments and the distribution of low birth weight in Chicago. *American Journal of Public Health, 87,* 597–603.

Roehling, M. (1999). Weight-based discrimination in employment: Psychological and legal aspects. *Personnel Psychology, 52,* 969–1016.

Rogers, I., Emmett, P., Baker, D., & Golding, J. (1998). Financial difficulties, smoking habits, composition of diet and birth weight in a population of pregnant women in the south-west of England. *European Journal of Clinical Nutrition, 52(4),* 251–60.

Rose, S. (1983). Differential rates of visual informational processing in full-term and pre-term infants. *Child Development, 54,* 11989–98.

Rosenbaum, E. (1997). Racial/ethnic differences in home ownership and housing quality. *Social Problems, 43,* 403–26.

Ross, C. (2000). Walking, exercising and smoking: Does neighborhood matter?
Social Science and Medicine, 5, 265–74.

Ruff, H., McCarton, C., Kurtzber, D., & Vaughan, H. (1984). Preterm infants'
manipulative exploration of objects. *Child Development, 55,* 116–73.

Ruggles, P. (1990). *Drawing the line: Alternative poverty measures and their
implications for public policy.* Washington, DC: Urban Institute Press.

Sachs, B., Fretts, R., Gardner, R., Hellersien, S., Wampler, N., & Wise, P. (1995).
The impact of extreme prematurity and congenital abnormalities on the inter-
pretation of international comparisons of infant mortality. *Obstetrics and
Gynecology, 85,* 941–46.

Sanderson, M., Williams, M., White, E., Daling, J., Holt, K., Malone, K., et al.
(1998). Validity and reliability of subject and mother reporting of perinatal
factors. *American Journal of Epidemiology, 147,* 136–140.

Sapolsky, R. (1993). Endrocrinology alfresco: Psycho-endocrine studies of wild
baboons. *Recent Progess in Hormone Research, 48,* 437–68.

Sapolsky, R. (1994). *Why zebras don't get ulcers: A guide to stress, stress related
diseases and coping.* New York: W. H. Freeman.

Saunder, P. (1996). *Poverty, income distribution and health: An Australian study*
(SPRC Reports and Proceedings No. 128). Sydney: University of New South
Wales, Social Policy Research Center.

Schachter, J., Lachin, J., & Wimberly, F. (1976). Newborn heart rate and blood
pressure: Relation to race and socioeconomic class. *Psychosomatic Medicine,
38,* 390–98.

Schloss, P., Smith, M., & Schloss, C. (2001). *Instructional methods for secondary students with learning and behavioral problems* (3rd ed.). Boston: Allyn
& Bacon.

Schneck, M., Sideras, K., Fox, R., & Dupuis, L. (1990). Low-income pregnancy, adolescents, and their infants: Dietary findings and health outcomes.
Journal of the American Dietetic Association, 90(4), 555–58.

Scholl, T., Hediger, M., & Vasilenko, P. (1989). Effects of early maturation of
fetal growth. *Annual Human Biology, 16,* 335–45.

Schribner, R., & Dwyer, J. (1989). Acculturation and low birthweight among
Latinos in the Hispanic HANES. *American Journal of Public Health, 79,*
1263–67.

Scott, D., & Spiker, D. (1989). Research on the sequelae of prematurity: Early
learning, early interventions and later outcomes. *Seminal Perinatology, 13,*
495–505.

Seidell, J. (1998). Societal and personal costs of obesity. *Experimental and Clinical Endocrinology and Diabetes, 106(2)(suppl),* 7–9.

Sepkowitz, S. (1995). International ranking of infant mortality and the U.S.:
Vital Statistics natality data collecting system-failures and success. *International Journal of Epidemiology, 24,* 583–88.

Sherraden, M., & Rossand, B. (1996). Poverty, family support and wellbeing of
infants: Mexican immigrant women and child bearing. *Journal of Sociology
and Social Welfare, 23(2),* 27–54.

Shmueli, A., & Cullen, M. (2000). Birth weight, maternal age, and education: New observations from Connecticut and Virginia. *Yale Journal of Biological Medicine, 72,* 245–58.

Showstack, J., Budetti, P., & Minkler, D. (1984). Factors associated with birth weight: An exploration of the roles of prenatal care and length of gestation. *American Journal of Public Health, 74,* 1003–8.

Smith, C. (1947). The effects of wartime starvation on pregnancy and its products. *American Journal of Obstetric Gynecology, 53,* 599–608.

Smith, D. (1998). *Introduction to special education: Teaching in an age of challenge* (3rd ed.). Boston: Allyn & Bacon.

Smith, J., Brooks-Gunn, J., & Klebanov, P. (1997). Consequences of living in poverty for young children's cognitive and verbal ability and early school achievement. In G. Duncan & J. Brooks-Gunn. (Eds.), *Consequences of growing up poor* (pp. 132–89). New York: Russell Sage Foundation.

Smith, S., & Dixon, R. (1995). Literacy concepts of low- and middle-class four year olds entering preschool. *Journal of Educational Research, 88,* 243–53.

Smith, T., Young, B., Bae, Y., Choy, S., & Alsalam, N. (1997). *The condition of education* (U.S. Department of Education, National Center for Educational Statistics Report No. 97-388). Washington, DC: U.S. Government Printing Office.

Sobal, J., & Stunkard, A. (1989). Socioeconomic status and obesity: A review of the literature. *Psychological Bulletin, 105,* 260–75.

Social Security Administration. (1998). *Food stamps and other nutritional programs* (Publication No. 05-10100). [Electronic version]. Washington, DC: Author. Retrieved September 25, 2001, from http://www.ssa.gov

Social Security Administration. (2000). *Benefits for children with disabilities* (SSA Publication No. 05-10026). [Electronic version]. Washington, DC: Author. Retrieved March 15, 2002, from www.ssa.gov/pubs/10026.html

Social Security Administration. (2002). SSI payment amounts, 1975–2002. Retrieved March 15, 2002, from http://www.ssa.gov/OACT/COLA/SSIamts .html

Soobader, M., & LeClere, F. (1999). Aggregation and the measurement of income inequality: Effects on morbidity. *Social Science and Medicine, 48,* 733–44.

Sorel, J., Rugland, D., Syme, S., & Davis, W. (1992). Educational status and blood pressure: The second national health and nutrition examination survey, 1976–1980. *American Journal of Epidemiology, 135,* 1339–48.

Sorensen, H., Sabroe, S., Olsen, J., Rothman, K., Gillman, M., & Fischer, P. (1997). Birth weight and cognitive function in young adult life: Historical cohort study. *British Medical Journal, 315,* 401–3.

Spiker, D., Ferguson, J., & Brooks-Gunn, J. (1993). Enhancing maternal interactive behavior and child social competence in low birth weight, preterm infants. *Child Development, 64,* 754–86.

SRI International. (1999). *National Early Intervention Longitudinal Study (NEILS): State-to-state variations in early intervention Systems* (Report prepared for the Office of Special Education Programs, U.S. Department of Education). Retrieved October 1, 2001, from http://www.sri.com/neils /reports/html

St. Peter, R., Newacheck, P., & Halfon, N. (1992). Access to care for poor children: Separate and unequal? *Journal of the American Medical Association, 267,* 2760–64.

Starfeild, B. (1991). Childhood morbidity: Comparisons, clusters, and trends. *Pediatrics, 88,* 519–26.

Starfield, B., Shapiro, S., Weiss, J., Liang, K., Ra, K., Paige, D., et al. (1991). Race, family income, and low birth weight. *American Journal of Epidemiology, 134,* 1167–74.

State Policy Documentation Project. (1999). Categorical eligibility: Pregnant women. Retrieved March 20, 2002, from http://www.spdp.prg/tanf/categorical/pregwom.pdf

State Policy Documentation Project. (1999). Financial eligibility for TANF cash assistance. Retrieved March 20, 2002, from http://www.spdp.org/tanf/financial/finansumm.htm

State Policy Documentation Project. (2000). Sanctions for non-compliance with work activities. Retrieved March 20, 2002, from http://www.spdp.org/tanf/sanctions.htm

State Policy Documentation Project. (2000). State policies regarding TANF work activities and requirements. Retrieved March 20, 2002, from http://www.spdp.org/tanf/sanctions/sanctions_findings.htm

Steckel, R. (1983). Height and per capita income. *Historical Methods, 16,* 1–7.

Stein, Z., Susser, M., Saegner, G., & Marrrolla, F. (1975). *Famine and human development: The Dutch hunger winter of 1944–1945.* New York: Oxford University Press.

Stellman, S., & Stellman, J. (1980). Health problems among 535 Vietnam veterans exposed to herbicides. *American Journal of Epidemiology, 112,* 444.

Stephan, N., & Gilman, S. (1991). Appropriating the idioms of science: The rejection of scientific racism. In D. LaCapra (Ed.), *The bonds of race: Perspectives on hegemony and resistance* (pp. 72–103). Ithaca, NY: Cornell University Press.

Stevens, J. (in press). Symbolic matter: DNA and other linguistic stuff. *Social Text.*

Stevens, R., & Stevens, R. (1974). *Welfare medicine in America: A case study of Medicaid.* New York: The Free Press.

Strauss, R. (2000). Adult functional outcome of those born small for gestational age: Twenty-six-year follow-up of the 1970 British birth cohort. *Journal of the American Medical Association, 283,* 625–31.

Strobino, D., Ensminger, M., Kim, Y., & Nanda, J. (1995). Mechanisms for maternal age differences in birth weight. *American Journal of Epidemiology, 142,* 504–14.

Stunkard, A. (1996). Socioeconomic status and obesity. *Origins and Consequences of Obesity, 201,* 174–87.

Sulloway, F. (1996). *Born to rebel: Birth order, family dynamics and creative lives.* New York: Pantheon Books.

Talan, J. (1998, December 22). Left-handed? Right-handed? Geneticist offers clues. *Newsday,* p. Z06.

Talbot, G., Goldstein, R., Nesbitt, T., Johnson, J., & Kay, H. (1997). Is size discordancy an indication for delivery of preterm twins? *American Journal of
Obstetric Gynecology, 177,* 1050–54.

TeKolste, K., & Bennett, F. (1987). The high-risk infant: Transitions in health,
development, and family during the first years of life. *Journal of Perinatology, 7,* 368–77.

Thomson, A. (2001, July 20). Homosexuality may be in the genes. *Toronto
Star,* p. 4.

Toner, R. (2002, February 1). Administration plans care of fetuses in a health
plan. [Electronic version]. *New York Times.* Retrieved February 1, 2002,
from http://www.nytimes.com

Troutt, D. (1993). The thin red line: How the poor still pay more. San Francisco Consumers Union of the United States, West Coast Regional Office.

U.S. Census Bureau (2000). American housing survey of the United States, 1999:
Table 2-1. Introductory characteristics—occupied units. Retrieved January
2002 from www.census.gov/hhes/www/housing/ahs/ahs99/ahs99.htm

U.S. Department of Agriculture. (1990, October). The savings in Medicaid
costs for newborns and their mothers from prenatal participation in the
WIC program, Volume 1 [Electronic Version]. Washington, DC: U.S. Government Printing Office. Retrieved October 2, 2001, from http://www.fns
.usda.gov/oane/MENU/Published/WIC/WIC.htm

U.S. Department of Agriculture. (1991, October). The savings in Medicaid
costs for newborns and their mothers from prenatal participation in the
WIC program, Addendum [Electronic Version]. Washington, DC: U.S. Government Printing Office. Retrieved October 2, 2001, from http://www.fns
.usda.gov/oane/MENU/Published/WIC/WIC.htm

U.S. Department of Agriculture. (1992, April). The savings in Medicaid costs
for newborns and their mothers from prenatal participation in the WIC
program, Volume 2. [Electronic Version]. Washington, DC: U.S. Government
Printing Office. Retrieved October 2, 2001, from http://www.fns.usda.gov
/oane/MENU/Published/WIC/WIC.htm

U.S. Department of Agriculture. (2000). WIC general analysis project: Profile
of WIC children. Retrieved September 23, 2001, from http://www.fns.usda
.gov/oane/MENU/published/WIC/FILES/profile.pdf

U.S. Department of Agriculture. (2000). *WIC participant and program characteristics, 1998* (Nutrition Assistance Program Report Series, Special Nutrition Programs, Report No. WIC-00-PC: 67-72). [Electronic Version]. Washington, DC: Author. (Retrieved September 23, 2001, from http://www.fns
.usda.gov/oane/MENU/Published/WIC/WIC.htm)

U.S. Department of Agriculture. (n.d.). WIC income eligibility criteria,
2001–2002. Retrieved September 20, 2001, from http://www.fns.usda.gov
/wic/incomeeligguidelines02-03.htm

U.S. Department of Education, Early Childhood Technical Assistance Center.
(2002). Overview to the Part C Program under IDEA. Retrieved October 1,
2001, from http://www.ectac.org

U.S. Department of Education. (1996). To assure the free appropriate public
education of all children with disabilities: 18th annual report to Congress

on the implementation of the Individuals with Disabilities Education Act. Retrieved October 1, 2001, from www.ed.gov/pubs/OSEP96AnlRpt/chap3 .html

U.S. Department of Education, Office of Special Education Programs. (2000). To assure the free appropriate public education of all children with disabilities: 22nd annual report to Congress on the implementation of the Individuals with Disabilities Education Act. Retrieved October 1, 2001, from http: //www.ed.gov/offices/OSERS/OSEP/products/OSEP2000AnIRpt/index.html

U.S. Department of Education, Office of Special Education Programs. (2002). Individuals with disabilities education act: Program-funded activities fiscal year 2001. Retrieved September 25, 2001, from http://www.ed.gov/offices /OSERS/OSEP/Programs/PFA2001/

U.S. General Accounting Office (1994, May). *Medicaid prenatal care: States improve access and enhance services but face new challenges* Washington, DC: U.S. Government Printing Office.

Vagero, D., & Illsley, R. (1995). Explaining health inequality: Beyond Black and Barker. *European Sociological Review, 11,* 219–41.

Vaughan, V., & Mkay, J. (1975). *Textbook of pediatrics.* Philadelphia: Saunders.

Vega, W., & Amaro, H. (1994). Latino outlook: Good health, uncertain prognosis. *Annual Review of Public Health, 15,* 39–67.

Ventura, S., Martin, J., Curtin, S., Mathews, T., & Park, M. (2000). Births: Final data for 1998. *National Vital Statistics Reports, 48(3).* Hyattsville, MA: National Center for Health Statistics.

Villermé, L. (1840). *Tableau d'etat physique et moral des ouvriers, Vol. 2.* Paris: Renouard.

Wang, X., Zuckerman, B., Coffman, G., & Corwin, M. (1995). Familial aggregation of low birth weight among whites and blacks in the United States. *New England Journal of Medicine, 333,* 1744–49.

Washington, V., & Bailey, U. (1995). *Project Head Start: Models and strategies for the twenty-first century.* New York: Garland.

Weaver, R. (2000). *Ending welfare as we know it.* Washington, DC: Brookings Institution Press.

Webb, R., & Shaw, N. (2001). Respiratory distress in heavier versus lighter twins. *Journal of Perinatal Medicine, 29,* 60–63.

West, C. (1993). *Race matters.* Boston: Beacon Press.

West, C., Adi, Y., & Pharoah, P. (1999). Fetal and infant death in mono- and dizygotic twins in England and Wales, 1982–1991. *Archive of Diseases in Childhood, Fetal and Neonatal Edition, 80,* F217–F220.

Widga, A., & Lewis, N. (1999). Defined, in-home prenatal nutrition intervention for low-income women. *Journal of the American Dietetic Association, 99(9),* 1058–62.

Wiener, G., Rider, R., Oppel, W., & Harper, P. (1968). Correlates of low birthweight: Psychological status at eight to ten years of age. *Pediatric Residence, 2,* 110.

Wilcox, A., & Russell, I. (1990). Why small black infants have a lower mortality rate than small white infants: The case for population-specific standards for birth weight. *Journal of Pediatrics, 116,* 7–10.

Wilkinson, R. (1986). Income inequality. In R. Wilkinson (Ed.), *Class and health: Research and longitudinal data* (pp. 1–20). London: Tavistock.

Wilkinson, R. (1992). Income distribution and life expectancy. *British Medical Journal, 304,* 165–68.

Wilkinson, R. (1996). *Unhealthy societies: The afflictions of inequality.* New York: Routledge.

Wilkinson, R. (Ed.). (1986). *Class and health: Research and longitudinal data.* London: Tavistock.

Will, M. [1984]. *Bridges from school to working life: OSERS programming for the transition of youth with disabilities* [policy report]. Washington DC: U.S. Department of Education, Office of Special Education and Rehabilitation Services.

Williams, D. (1992). Black-white difference in blood pressure: The role of social factors. *Ethnicity and Disease, 2,* 126–41.

Williams, D. (1994). The concept of race in health services research, 1966–1990. *Health Services Research, 29,* 261–74.

Williams, D., & Collins, C. (1995). U.S. socioeconomic and racial differences in health: Patterns and explanations. *Annual Review of Sociology, 21,* 349–86.

Williams, D., Lavizzo-Maourey, R., & Warren, R. (1994). The concept of race and health status in America. *Public Health Reports, 109,* 26–42.

Williams, M., & O'Brien, W. (1997). Twins, asymmetric growth restriction, and perinatal morbidity. *Journal of Perinatology, 17,* 468–72.

Wilson, W. (1978). *The declining significance of race and changing American institutions.* Chicago: University of Chicago Press.

Wolff, E. (2000). Recent trends in wealth ownership, 1983–1998. The Jerome Levy Institute Working Paper no. 300.

Yalcin, H., Zorlu, C., Lembet, A., Ozden, S., & Gokmen, O. (1998). The significance of birth weight difference in discordant twins: A level to standardize? *Acta Obstetrica Gyneologica Scandinavia, 77,* 28–31.

Zigler, E., & Styfco, S. (1993). *Head Start and beyond: A national plan for extended childhood intervention.* New Haven, CT: Yale University Press.

Zill, N., Moore, K., Smith, E., Stief, T., & Corio, M. (1991).*The life circumstances and development on children in welfare families: A profile based on national survey data.* Washington, DC: Child Trends.

Index

Compositor:	Michael Bass Associates
Indexer:	Ron Strauss
Text:	10/13 Sabon
Display:	Sabon
Printer and binder:	The Maple-Vail Book Manufacturing Group